D0641688

The Addiction Casebook

The Addiction Casebook

Edited by

Petros Levounis, M.D., M.A.

Abigail J. Herron, D.O.

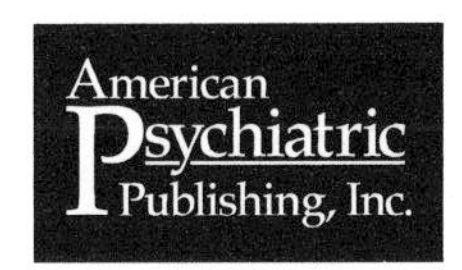

Washington, DC
London, England

Note: The authors have worked to ensure that all information in this book is accurate at the time of publication and consistent with general psychiatric and medical standards, and that information concerning drug dosages, schedules, and routes of administration is accurate at the time of publication and consistent with standards set by the U.S. Food and Drug Administration and the general medical community. As medical research and practice continue to advance, however, therapeutic standards may change. Moreover, specific situations may require a specific therapeutic response not included in this book. For these reasons and because human and mechanical errors sometimes occur, we recommend that readers follow the advice of physicians directly involved in their care or the care of a member of their family.

Books published by American Psychiatric Publishing (APP) represent the findings, conclusions, and views of the individual authors and do not necessarily represent the policies and opinions of APP or the American Psychiatric Association.

If you would like to buy between 25 and 99 copies of this or any other American Psychiatric Publishing title, you are eligible for a 20% discount; please contact Customer Service at appi@psych.org or 800-368-5777. If you wish to buy 100 or more copies of the same title, please e-mail us at bulksales@psych.org for a price quote.

Copyright © 2014 American Psychiatric Association
ALL RIGHTS RESERVED

Manufactured in the United States of America on acid-free paper
18 17 16 15 14 5 4 3 2 1
First Edition

Typeset in Trade Gothic and Minion Pro.

American Psychiatric Publishing

A Division of American Psychiatric Association
1000 Wilson Boulevard
Arlington, VA 22209-3901
www.appi.org

Library of Congress Cataloging-in-Publication Data
The addiction casebook / [edited by] Petros Levounis, Abigail J. Herron. — First edition.

p. ; cm.

Includes bibliographical references and index.

ISBN 978-1-58562-458-4 (pbk. : alk. paper)

I. Levounis, Petros, editor of compilation. II. Herron, Abigail J., 1977– editor of compilation. III. American Psychiatric Association, issuing body.

[DNLM: 1. Substance-Related Disorders—Case Reports. 2. Behavior, Addictive—Case Reports. WM 270]

RC564.29

362.29--dc23 2013041547

British Library Cataloguing in Publication Data
A CIP record is available from the British Library.

Contents

Part I. Introduction

Part II. Substance-Related Disorders

Contributors

Michael Ascher, M.D.
Fellow, Department of Psychiatry, Hospital of the University of Pennsylvania Addictions Fellowship Program, Philadelphia Veterans Administration Medical Center, Philadelphia, Pennsylvania

Robbie Bahl, M.D.
Medical Director, Cedar Hill Hospital, Portland, Oregon

Silvia Bernardi, M.D.
Postdoctoral Residency Fellow, Department of Psychiatry, New York State Psychiatric Institute/Columbia University, New York, New York

Saadiq J. Bey, M.S.W., CASAC, ICADC
Research Assistant, AIDS Community Research Initiative of America, New York, New York

Carlos Blanco, M.D., Ph.D.
Professor of Clinical Psychiatry, Department of Psychiatry, New York State Psychiatric Institute/Columbia University, New York, New York

Timothy K. Brennan, M.D., M.P.H.
Associate Director, Fellowship in Addiction Medicine and Attending Physician, Addiction Institute of New York, New York, New York

Faye Chao, M.D.
Unit Chief, Inpatient Service, Addiction Institute of New York, St. Luke's–Roosevelt Hospital Center, New York, New York

Elias Dakwar, M.D.
Assistant Professor of Clinical Psychiatry, Department of Psychiatry, New York State Psychiatric Institute/Columbia University, New York, New York

Erin M. Delker, M.P.H.
New York State Psychiatric Institute, New York, New York

Deborah S. Hasin, Ph.D.
Department of Psychiatry, College of Physicians and Surgeons and Department of Epidemiology, Mailman School of Public Health, Columbia University; New York State Psychiatric Institute, New York, New York

Abigail J. Herron, D.O.
Director, Fellowship in Addiction Medicine, and Acting Medical Director, Addiction Institute of New York, St. Luke's–Roosevelt Hospital Center, New York, New York

Claudie H. Jimenez, M.D., M.S.
Medical Director, Chemical Dependency Services, Harlem East Life Plan, New York, New York

Gary P. Katzman, M.D.
Clinical Assistant Professor, Icahn School of Medicine at Mount Sinai, New York, New York

Steven Joseph Lee, M.D.

Petros Levounis, M.D., M.A.
Chair, Department of Psychiatry, Rutgers New Jersey Medical School, Newark, New Jersey

Glenn Occhiogrosso, M.D.
Unit Chief, Inpatient Detoxification Service, Kings County Hospital Center, Brooklyn, New York

Mayumi Okuda, M.D.
Postdoctoral Residency Fellow, Department of Psychiatry, New York State Psychiatric Institute/Columbia University, New York, New York

Aykut Ozden, M.D.
Clinical Assistant Professor of Psychiatry, Columbia University College of Physicians and Surgeons; Director, Comprehensive Assessment Center, Department of Psychiatry, St. Luke's–Roosevelt Hospital Center, New York, New York

Joe Ruggiero, Ph.D.
Assistant Clinical Director, Addiction Institute of New York; Director, Crystal Clear Project, St. Luke's–Roosevelt Hospital Center, New York, New York

Shaneel Shah, M.D.
Child and Adolescent Psychiatry Fellow, Child and Adolescent Psychiatry Division, Department of Psychiatry, St. Luke's–Roosevelt Hospital Center, New York, New York

Susan D. Whitley, M.D.
Director of Chemical Dependency Services, Kings County Hospital Center; Clinical Assistant Professor of Psychiatry and Family Medicine, State University of New York Downstate, Brooklyn, New York

Disclosure of Interests

The following contributors have indicated that they have no financial interests or other affiliations that represent or could appear to represent a competing interest with their contributions to this book:

Michael Ascher, M.D.; Robbie Bahl, M.D., Saadiq J. Bey, M.S.W., CASAC, ICADC; Timothy K. Brennan, M.D., M.P.H.; Faye Chao, M.D.; Elias Dakwar, M.D.; Deborah S. Hasin, Ph.D.; Abigail J. Herron, D.O.; Claudie H. Jimenez, M.D., M.S.; Gary P. Katzman, M.D.; Steven Joseph Lee, M.D.; Petros Levounis, M.D., M.A.; Mayumi Okuda, M.D.; Aykut Ozden, M.D.; Joe Ruggiero, Ph.D.; Shaneel Shah, M.D.; Susan D. Whitley, M.D.

Preface

FEW illnesses come with more stigma and misunderstanding than the addictions. The majority of our patients who have substance use disorders are not properly diagnosed and do not receive adequate medical care. Yet working with these patients is both scientifically fascinating and immensely rewarding.

Although this casebook is far from complete in covering the breadth and depth of our current knowledge in the diagnosis and treatment of substance use and other addictive disorders, we hope that it will provide the fundamental tools for working with the substance-using patient in the hospital, the clinic, and the community.

The book begins with an introductory chapter that outlines the progression of our thinking in terms of psychiatric diagnosis as we move from DSM-IV-TR (American Psychiatric Association 2000) to DSM-5 (American Psychiatric Association 2013). This first chapter is different in tone and format from the rest of the book and explains the reasoning behind the change in criteria sets and the broadening of the concept of addictive disorders to include the behavioral addictions. It is followed by 12 case studies with assessment tools and treatment recommendations. Each case study introduces a patient with an addiction DSM-5 diagnosis (except for the last chapter on problematic Internet use) followed by a discussion that illustrates common ways of working with addicted patients. An additional goal of the book is to show clinicians who have little experience in this area the intersection of addiction with other psychiatric diagnoses.

This casebook has been a collaboration of three generations of addiction specialists. We have invited our peers, as well as our mentors and our students, to join us in formulating the most salient ideas and suggestions that we have found helpful for treating people who are dealing with substance use and other addictions. We are indebted to them for their great insights and clinical wisdom. We are also deeply grateful to our patients, colleagues, friends, and families for their inspiration and support throughout the writing of this book. Finally, a special thanks goes to our husbands, Lukas and Donald, whose affectionate patience with our writing schedules can only be explained by true love and even truer hope for *Addiction Casebook*–free summer weekends.

Petros Levounis, M.D., M.A.
Abigail J. Herron, D.O.
June 2013

References

American Psychiatric Association: Diagnostic and Statistical Manual of Mental Disorders, 4th Edition, Text Revision. Washington, DC, American Psychiatric Association, 2000

American Psychiatric Association: Diagnostic and Statistical Manual of Mental Disorders, 5th Edition. Washington, DC, American Psychiatric Association, 2013

PART I

INTRODUCTION

CHAPTER 1

DSM-5 Criteria for Substance Use Disorders: Recommendations and Rationale

Deborah S. Hasin, Ph.D.
Erin M. Delker, M.P.H.

SINCE publication of DSM-IV in 1994 (American Psychiatric Association 1994), the DSM approach to substance use disorders (SUDs) has come under scrutiny. Strengths were identified (notably, reliability and validity of dependence), but concerns have also arisen. The DSM-5 SUD Workgroup (Charles O'Brien, M.D., Ph.D.; Marc Auriacombe, M.D.; Guilherme Borges, Sc.D.; Kathleen Bucholz, Ph.D.; Alan Budney, Ph.D.; Wilson Compton, M.D., M.P.E.; Thomas Crowley, M.D.; Bridget F. Grant, Ph.D., Ph.D.; Deborah S. Hasin, Ph.D.; Walter Ling, M.D.; Nancy M. Petry, Ph.D.; and Marc Schuckit, M.D.) considered these issues and recommended revisions for DSM-5 (American Psychiatric Association 2013). General concerns included whether to retain the division into two main disorders (dependence and abuse), whether SUD criteria should be added or removed, and whether an appropriate SUD severity

---

Disclaimer: The views and opinions expressed in this chapter are those of the authors and should not be construed to represent the views of any of the sponsoring organizations or agencies or the U.S. government.

indicator could be identified. Specific issues included possible addition of withdrawal syndromes for several substances; alignment of nicotine criteria with those for other substances; addition of biomarkers; and inclusion of nonsubstance, behavioral "addictions." In this chapter we present the major issues and evidence considered by the workgroup, which included literature reviews and extensive new data analyses. Workgroup recommendations for DSM-5 revisions included combining abuse and dependence criteria into a single SUD on the basis of consistent findings from more than 200,000 participants, dropping legal problems and adding craving, adding cannabis and caffeine withdrawal, aligning nicotine criteria with other disorders, and moving gambling disorder to the chapter formerly reserved only for substance-related disorders. The proposed changes overcome many problems, although future studies will be needed to address issues for which fewer data were available.

The *Diagnostic and Statistical Manual of Mental Disorders* (DSM) is the standard classification of mental disorders used for clinical, research, policy, and reimbursement purposes in the United States and elsewhere. DSM therefore has widespread importance and influence on how disorders are diagnosed, treated, and investigated. Since its first publication in 1952, DSM has been reviewed and revised four times; the criteria in the previous version, DSM-IV-TR, were first published in 1994. Since then, knowledge about psychiatric disorders, including substance use disorders, has advanced greatly. To take the advances into account, a new version, DSM-5, was published in 2013. The shift to Arabic numerals in DSM-5 is a departure from the traditional use of roman numerals applied in previous versions of the manual (e.g., DSM-IV-TR). This change in nomenclature will clearly denote any future changes to the criteria. It also allows for more frequent and responsive adjustments to DSM as developing research elucidates ways to improve diagnoses.

In 2007, the American Psychiatric Association convened a multidisciplinary team of experts, the DSM-5 SUD Workgroup, to identify strengths and problems in the DSM-IV approach to SUDs and to recommend improvements for DSM-5. Using a set of 2006 reviews (Saunders and Schuckit 2006) as a starting point, the workgroup noted weaknesses, highlighted gaps in knowledge, identified data sets to investigate possible solutions, encouraged or conducted analyses to fill knowledge gaps, monitored relevant new publications, and formulated interim recommendations for proposed changes. The workgroup elicited input on proposed changes through commentary, expert advisors, the DSM-5 Web site (which received 520 comments on SUDs), and presentations at more than 30 professional meetings. In this chapter we present problems identified with DSM-IV and revisions for DSM-5 to provide an improved approach to SUDs.

Overarching Issues

Should Abuse and Dependence Be Kept as Two Separate Diagnoses?

The DSM-IV criteria for substance abuse and dependence are shown in Figure 1–1. Dependence was diagnosed when three or more dependence criteria were met. Among patients with no dependence diagnosis, abuse was diagnosed when at least one abuse criterion was met. The criteria for dependence were consistently shown to be highly reliable and valid (Hasin et al. 2006). However, some aspects of the DSM-IV approach pertaining to the diagnosis of abuse and the stipulated hierarchical relationship of abuse and dependence were problematic.

First, when diagnosed hierarchically according to DSM-IV, abuse had inconsistent reliability and validity. When analyzed without regard to dependence, the abuse criteria test-retest reliability improved considerably. Second, by definition, a syndrome requires more than one symptom, but nearly half of all abuse cases were diagnosed with only one criterion, most often hazardous use (Hasin et al. 1999). Third, although *abuse* is often assumed to be milder than *dependence,* some abuse criteria indicate clinically severe problems, such as substance-related failure to fulfill major responsibilities. In addition, the case of *diagnostic orphans* (Pollock and Martin 1999), with two dependence and no abuse criteria, is potentially more serious than abuse but was ineligible for a diagnosis.

Fourth, factor analyses of dependence and abuse criteria (ignoring the DSM-IV hierarchy) showed that the criteria formed one factor (Krueger et al. 2004) or two very highly correlated factors (Grant et al. 2007), suggesting that the criteria should be combined into a single disorder. Finally, item response analysis (IRT), an extension of factor analysis, suggested that the criteria intermixed across a spectrum range of latent trait severity, invalidating the DSM-IV established hierarchical relationship of abuse and dependence. Abuse criteria ranged from common but low severity (hazardous use) to rare but high severity (neglect of major roles to use). Collectively, this large body of evidence supported removing the distinction between abuse and dependence.

Decision: For DSM-5, combine abuse and dependence criteria into one disorder (Figure 1–1), with two additional changes indicated in the following two sections.

Should Any of the Diagnostic Criteria Be Dropped?

If any criteria could be dropped while retaining diagnostic accuracy, the set would be easier to use in clinical practice. The workgroup considered whether legal problems should be dropped. Reasons to drop legal problems included very low prevalence in adults and little added information in diagnosis. Some clinicians were concerned that dropping legal problems as a criterion would leave certain patients undiagnosed, an issue specifically addressed among heavy alcohol, cannabis, cocaine, and/or heroin users in methadone and dual-diagnosis psychiatric settings (Hasin et al. 2012). None of these patients reported substance-related legal problems as their only criterion or "lost" a DSM-5 SUD diagnosis without this criterion. Thus, legal problems are not a useful SUD criterion, although such problems may be an important treatment focus in some settings.

Decision: Drop legal problems as a DSM-5 diagnostic criterion.

Should Any Criteria Be Added?

If new criteria increase diagnostic accuracy, the set would be improved through their addition. The workgroup considered adding craving as a criterion. Support for craving as a SUD criterion comes indirectly from behavioral, imaging, pharmacology, and genetics studies. Craving is included among the dependence criteria in the International Classification of Diseases, 10th Revision (ICD-10; World Health Organization 1993), so adding craving to DSM-5 would increase consistency between the nosologies.

In previous studies, craving was measured with questions regarding a strong desire or urge to use the substance or such a strong desire to use that one could not think of anything else. Although some studies suggest that craving is redundant with other criteria (Casey et al. 2012) and the psychometric benefit is equivocal, clinicians expressed enthusiasm about adding it to the criteria because craving may become a biological treatment target (a nonpsychometric perspective).

Decisions: Add craving to the DSM-5 SUD criteria (Figure 1–1) as *craving or a strong desire or urge to use* the substance. Encourage further research on the role of craving among SUD criteria.

What Should Be the Diagnostic Threshold?

Although SUD criteria represent a dimensional condition with no natural threshold, determining a binary (yes or no) diagnostic decision is often useful. The workgroup sought a threshold for DSM-5 SUDs that would yield the best agreement with the prevalence of DSM-IV substance abuse and dependence disorders combined. Agreement with DSM-IV diagnoses was maximized with the threshold of ≥2 criteria, so it was selected (Table 1–1).

The professional and lay press (Urbina 2012) have expressed concerns that the threshold of ≥2 criteria is too low for several reasons (e.g., it may produce an

	DSM-IV abuse[a]		DSM-IV dependence[b]		DSM-5 SUD[c]	
Hazardous use	X		-		X	
Social/interpersonal problems related to use	X	≥1 criterion	-		X	
Neglect of major roles to use	X		-		X	
Legal problems	X		-		-	
Withdrawal[d]	-		X		X	
Tolerance	-		X		X	≥2 criteria
Use larger amounts/longer	-		X		X	
Repeated attempts to quit/control use	-		X	≥3 criteria	X	
Much time spent using	-		X		X	
Physical/psychological problems related to use	-		X		X	
Activities given up to use	-		X		X	
Craving	-		X		X	

FIGURE 1–1. DSM-IV and DSM-5 criteria for substance use disorders (SUDs).

[a]One or more abuse criteria within a 12-month period *and* no dependence diagnosis; applicable to all substances except nicotine, for which DSM-IV abuse criteria were not given.

[b]Three or more dependence criteria within a 12-month period.

[c]Two or more SUD criteria within a 12-month period.

[d]Withdrawal not included for cannabis, inhalant, and hallucinogen disorders in DSM-IV; cannabis withdrawal was added in DSM-5.

TABLE 1–1. Agreement between DSM-IV abuse/dependence and DSM-5 SUDs at different diagnostic thresholds

	Sample size	Prevalence	Kappa
NESARC			
Drinkers, last 12 months[a]	20,836		
DSM-IV alcohol		.10	
DSM-5, ≥2 criteria		.11	0.73
DSM-5, ≥3 criteria		.06	0.73
COGA nonproband adults			
Drinkers, lifetime	6,673		
DSM-IV alcohol		.43	
DSM-5, ≥2 criteria		.43	0.80
DSM-5, ≥3 criteria		.32	0.74
Cannabis users, lifetime	4,569		
DSM-IV cannabis		.35	
DSM-5, ≥2 criteria		.33	0.82
DSM-5, ≥3 criteria		.26	0.75
Cross-national emergency rooms			
Drinkers, last 12 months[a]	3,191		
DSM-IV alcohol		.21	
DSM-5, ≥2 criteria		.21	0.80
DSM-5, ≥3 criteria		.15	0.79
Metropolitan clinical sample (*N*=663)			
Drinkers, last 12 months[a]	534		
DSM-IV current alcohol		46.9	
DSM-5, ≥2 criteria		48.7	0.94
DSM-5, ≥3 criteria		45.7	0.96
DSM-5, ≥4 criteria		42.8	0.92
Cannabis users, last 12 months[a]	340		
DSM-IV cannabis		21.1	
DSM-5, ≥2 criteria		19.6	0.85
DSM-5, ≥3 criteria		16.4	0.83
DSM-5, ≥4 criteria		13.4	0.73
Cocaine users, last 12 months[a]	483		
DSM-IV cocaine		52.9	
DSM-5, ≥2 criteria		54.5	0.93

TABLE 1–1. Agreement between DSM-IV abuse/dependence and DSM-5 SUDs at different diagnostic thresholds *(continued)*

	Sample size	Prevalence	Kappa
DSM-5, ≥3 criteria		51.7	0.96
DSM-5, ≥4 criteria		48.9	0.93
Heroin users, last 12 months[a]	364		
DSM-IV heroin		40.0	
DSM-5, ≥2 criteria		41.6	0.95
DSM-5, ≥3 criteria		39.2	0.97
DSM-5, ≥4 criteria		36.5	0.96

Note. COGA=Collaborative Study on the Genetics of Alcoholism; NESARC=National Epidemiologic Survey on Alcohol and Related Conditions.
[a]Any use within prior 12 months.

overly heterogeneous group, or patients at low severity levels are not "true" cases). These understandable concerns were weighed against the competing need to identify all cases meriting intervention, including milder cases, such as those in primary care. Table 1–1 shows that a concern that "millions more" would be diagnosed with the DSM-5 threshold (Urbina 2012) is unfounded if DSM-5 SUD criteria are assessed and decision rules are followed (rather than assigning a SUD diagnosis to any substance user). Additional concerns about the threshold should be addressed by the severity indicators (see the section "How Should Severity Be Represented?"), which clearly indicate that cases vary in severity.

An important exception to making a diagnosis of DSM-5 SUD with two criteria pertains to supervised use of psychoactive substances for medical purposes, including stimulants; cocaine; opioids; nitrous oxide; sedative, hypnotic, or anxiolytic drugs; and cannabis in some jurisdictions. These substances can produce tolerance and/or withdrawal as normal physiological adaptations when used appropriately for supervised medical purposes. With a threshold of ≥2 criteria, these criteria could lead to invalid SUD diagnoses even with no other criteria met. Under these conditions, tolerance and withdrawal in the absence of other criteria do not indicate an SUD and should not be diagnosed as such.

Decision: Set the diagnostic threshold for DSM-5 SUDs at ≥2 criteria.

How Should Severity Be Represented?

The DSM-5 task force asked workgroups for severity indicators (mild, moderate, and severe) of diagnoses. Many severity indicators are possible (e.g., levels of use, impairment, comorbidity); the workgroup sought a simple, parsimonious approach. A count of the criteria themselves serves this purpose well because as the count increases, so does the likelihood of SUD risk factors and consequences.

Decisions: Use a criteria count as an overall severity indicator. Use two to three, four to five, and more than six criteria to indicate mild, moderate, and severe disorders, respectively.

Specifiers

Physiological Specifier

DSM-IV included a specifier for *physiological* cases, that is, those manifesting tolerance and/or withdrawal, a carryover from DSM-III. The predictive value of this specifier was inconsistent. Further, the specifier was unused outside of studies investigating its validity.

Decision: Eliminate the physiological specifier in DSM-5.

Course Specifiers

In DSM-IV, six course specifiers for *dependence* were provided. Four of these pertained to the time frame and completeness of remission, and two pertained to extenuating circumstances.

Completeness and Time Frame of Remission. In DSM-IV, these course specifiers were complex and little used. To simplify, the workgroup eliminated partial remission and divided the time frame into two categories, *early* and *sustained. Early remission* indicates a period ≥ 3 but < 12 months with no DSM-5 SUD criteria other than craving. Data indicate better outcomes for patients retained in treatment for at least 3 months (Hubbard et al. 2009). *Sustained remission* indicates a period lasting ≥ 12 months with no DSM-5 SUD criteria other than craving. Craving is an exception because it can persist long into remission.

The workgroup noted that many clinical studies define remission and relapse in terms of substance use per se, not DSM criteria. The workgroup did not do this to remain consistent with DSM-IV criteria and because the criteria focus on substance-related difficulties, not the extent of use, for the reasons discussed in the section "Should Any Criteria Be Added?" Also, lack of consensus on the level of use associated with a good outcome (Tiffany et al. 2012) complicates substance use as a course specifier for the disorder.

Decisions: Define early remission as ≥ 3 to < 12 months without SUD criteria (except craving) and sustained remission as ≥ 12 months without SUD criteria (except craving).

Extenuating Circumstances. *In a controlled environment* was unchanged from DSM-IV. DSM-IV included *on agonist therapy,* such as methadone or unspecified partial agonists or agonist/antagonists. To update this category, DSM-5 replaced it with *on maintenance therapy* and provided specific examples.

Decision: Update the maintenance therapy category with examples: agonists (e.g., methadone, buprenorphine), antagonists (e.g., naltrexone), and tobacco cessation medication (bupropion, varenicline).

Could the Definitions of Substance-Induced Mental Disorders Be Improved?

Substance use and mental disorders frequently co-occur, complicating diagnosis because many symptoms (e.g., insomnia) are criteria for intoxication or withdrawal syndromes and also for other mental disorders. In DSM-IV, primary mental disorders were diagnosed if they began prior to substance use or persisted >4 weeks after cessation of acute withdrawal or severe intoxication. DSM-IV substance-induced mental disorders were defined as occurring during periods of substance intoxication or withdrawal or remitting within 4 weeks thereafter. Symptoms listed both for the relevant disorder *and* for intoxication or withdrawal from substances used were counted toward the substance-induced mental disorder only if they exceeded the expected severity of intoxication or withdrawal.

DSM-IV substance-induced mental disorders were diagnostically challenging because of the absence of minimum duration and symptom requirements and guidelines on when symptoms exceeded expected severity for intoxication or withdrawal. Also, the term *primary* was confusing, implying a time sequence or diagnostic hierarchy. Research showed that DSM-IV substance-induced mental disorders could be diagnosed reliably and validly by standardizing procedures to determine when symptoms were greater than expected (although these were complex) and, importantly, by requiring the same duration and symptom criteria as the corresponding primary mental disorder. These concerns led to a flexible approach that reversed the DSM-IV standardization.

Decisions: 1) For a diagnosis of substance-induced mental disorder, add a criterion that the disorder resembles the full criteria for the relevant disorder. 2) Remove the requirement that symptoms exceed expected intoxication or withdrawal symptoms. 3) Specify that the substance must be pharmacologically capable of producing the psychiatric symptoms. 4) Change the wording *primary* to *independent.* 5) Adjust the name from *substance-induced* to *substance/medication-induced* disorders because the latter were included in both DSM-IV and DSM-5 criteria but were not noted in the names of the disorders in DSM-IV.

Could Biomarkers Be Utilized in Making SUD Diagnoses?

The workgroup considered the following biomarkers: 1) pharmacokinetic measures of the psychoactive substances or their metabolites, 2) genetic markers, and 3) brain imaging indicators of brain structure and function. Many measures of drugs and associated metabolites in blood, urine, sweat, saliva, hair, and breath can indicate whether a substance was taken within a limited recent time window but cannot be used to diagnose SUDs. Emerging genetic and brain imaging research is beneficial to identifying predictors of SUDs but is inconclusive for determining diagnoses. Continued research in this area is important.

Decision: Biomarkers are not included.

Should Polysubstance Dependence Be Retained?

In DSM-IV, polysubstance dependence allowed diagnosis of multiple-substance users who failed to meet dependence criteria for any one substance but had ≥3 dependence criteria collectively across substances. The category was often misunderstood as dependence on multiple substances and was little used (Schuckit et al. 2001). With the new threshold for DSM-5 SUD (≥2 criteria), the category became irrelevant.

Decision: Eliminate polysubstance dependence.

Substance-Specific Issues

Should Caffeine, Cannabis, Inhalant, and Hallucinogen Withdrawal Disorders Be Added, and If So, Should These Withdrawal Syndromes Be Added to SUD Criteria for the Relevant Substances?

Caffeine

In DSM-IV, caffeine withdrawal was included as a research diagnosis to encourage further study. Accumulated evidence from preclinical and clinical studies supports the reliability, validity, pharmacological specificity, and clinical significance of caffeine withdrawal. The workgroup proposed modifying the DSM-IV research criteria so that in DSM-5 diagnosis would require three or more of these symptoms: 1) headache; 2) fatigue or drowsiness; 3) dysphoric mood or irritability; 4) difficulty concentrating; and 5) nausea, vomiting, or muscle pain/stiffness (Juliano et al. 2012). Clinical and epidemiological studies with larger samples and more diverse populations are needed to determine prevalence, establish a consistent set of diagnostic criteria, and better evaluate the clinical significance of a caffeine use disorder. These studies should address test-retest reliability and antecedent, concurrent, and predictive validity.

Decisions: Add caffeine withdrawal disorder and include caffeine use disorder in Section III, "Conditions for Further Study."

Cannabis

Cannabis withdrawal was not included in DSM-IV because of lack of evidence. Since then, the reliability and validity of cannabis withdrawal have been demonstrated in preclinical, clinical, and epidemiological studies. The syndrome has a transient course after cessation of cannabis use (Copersino et al. 2006) and pharmacological specificity. Cannabis withdrawal is reported by up to one-third of regular users in the general population and by 50%–95% of heavy users in treatment or research studies (Copersino et al. 2006). The clinical significance of cannabis withdrawal is demonstrated by use of cannabis or other substances to relieve it, its association with difficulty quitting (Copersino et al. 2006), and worse treatment outcomes associated with greater withdrawal severity.

Decisions: Add cannabis withdrawal disorder. Include withdrawal as a criterion for cannabis use disorder.

Inhalants and Hallucinogens

Although some support exists for adding withdrawal syndromes for inhalants and 3,4-methylenedioxy-*N*-methylamphetamine (ecstasy), literature and expert consultation suggested that evidence remained insufficient to include these in DSM-5 but that further study is warranted.

Decision: Further research on inhalant withdrawal and hallucinogen withdrawal is needed.

Could the Nicotine Criteria Be Aligned With the Diagnostic Criteria for the Other SUDs?

Concerns about DSM-IV-defined nicotine dependence (ND) include 1) utility of some criteria, 2) ability to predict treatment outcome, and 3) low prevalence in smokers (Budney and Hughes 2006).

Smoking researchers widely regard craving as a dependence and relapse indicator (Benowitz 2010). Increasing disapproval of smoking and wider smoking restrictions (Colgrove et al. 2011) suggest improved face validity of *continued tobacco use despite having persistent or recurrent social or interpersonal problems* and smoking-related *failure to fulfill major role obligations* as criteria for tobacco use disorder. Smoking is highly associated with fire-related and other mortality (e.g., unintentional injuries, vehicle crashes) (Benowitz 2010), suggesting the applicability of *hazardous use.*

In IRT analyses, the 11 criteria formed a unidimensional (one factor) latent trait intermixed across the severity spectrum, significantly increasing information over a model with DSM-IV ND criteria only. The proposed tobacco use disorder criteria (individually and as a set) were strongly associated with a panel of validators, including smoking quantity and smoking shortly after awakening (Shmulewitz et al. 2013). The tobacco use disorder criteria were more discriminating than the DSM-IV ND criteria (Shmulewitz et al. 2013) and produced a higher prevalence than DSM-IV ND criteria, addressing a DSM-IV concern (Hughes et al. 2006).

Decision: Align DSM-5 criteria for tobacco use disorder with criteria for the other SUDs.

Should Neurobehavioral Disorder Associated With Prenatal Alcohol Exposure Be Added?

Neurobehavioral disorder associated with prenatal alcohol exposure (ND-PAE) results when in utero alcohol exposure acts as a neurobehavioral teratogen (Guerri et al. 2009). Key features include neurocognitive and behavioral impairments diagnosed through standardized psychological or educational testing, caregiver or teacher questionnaires, medical records, reports of the patient and/or a knowledgeable informant, or clinician observation. Prenatal alcohol exposure can be determined by maternal self-report, others' reported observations of maternal drinking during the pregnancy, and/or documentation in medical or other records.

ND-PAE was not included in DSM-IV. Proposed diagnostic guidelines allow ND-PAE diagnosis regardless of the facial dysmorphology required to diagnose fetal alcohol syndrome. Many clinical experts support the diagnosis (National Institute on Alcohol Abuse and Alcoholism 2011), and clinical need is suggested by substantial misdiagnosis, leading to unmet treatment need (National Institute on Alcohol Abuse and Alcoholism 2011). However, more information is needed on ND-PAE before it can be included in the main manual.

Decision: Include ND-PAE in Section III, "Conditions for Further Study."

Issues Not Related to Substances

Should Gambling Disorder and Other Putative Behavioral "Addictions" Be Added to the Substance Disorders Chapter?

Gambling

In DSM-IV, pathological gambling (PG) is in the section "Impulse-Control Disorders Not Elsewhere Classified." PG is comorbid with substance use disorders

(Kessler et al. 2008) and is similar to SUDs in some symptom presentations, biological dysfunction, genetic liability, and treatment approaches. In DSM-5, the name was changed to *gambling disorder* because the term *pathological* is pejorative and redundant. The criterion *illegal acts... to finance gambling* was removed for the same reasons that legal problems were removed from SUDs. The diagnostic threshold was reduced to ≥4 criteria to improve classification accuracy (Denis et al. 2012). A further reduction in the threshold was considered, but this greatly increased prevalence without evidence for diagnostic improvement. Future work should explore whether gambling disorder can be assessed using parallel criteria to those for SUDs (Denis et al. 2012).

Other Nonsubstance Disorders

The workgroup consulted outside experts and reviewed literature on other potential nonsubstance behaviors, such as Internet gaming and shopping. This review included more than 200 publications on Internet gaming addiction, mostly Asian case reports and/or case series of articles studying young males. Despite the large literature, additional studies are needed to ascertain the unique characteristics of the disorder, cross-cultural reliability and validity data of diagnostic criteria, prevalence in representative samples, natural history, and potentially associated biological factors. Research on other "behavioral addictions" is even more preliminary.

Decisions: Include gambling disorder in the SUD chapter, with changes noted above. Add Internet gaming disorder to Section III.

Should the Name of the Chapter Be Changed?

With the addition of gambling disorder to the chapter, a change in the title was necessary. The Board of Trustees assigned the title "Substance-Related and Addictive Disorders" despite tension over the terms *addiction* and *dependence.*

Present Status and Future Directions

Beginning in 2007, the SUD workgroup conducted and published analyses, formulated new criteria, and presented the criteria widely for input. Implementing the 11 DSM-5 SUD criteria in research and clinical assessment should be easier than implementing the 11 DSM-IV criteria for substance abuse and dependence because now only one disorder is involved instead of two hierarchical disorders. A checklist can aid in covering all criteria. Eventually, reducing the number of criteria to diagnose SUDs would aid further in implementation, which future studies should address.

Many studies showed that DSM-IV dependence was reliable and valid (Hasin et al. 2006), suggesting that major components of the DSM-5 SUD criteria are reliable as well. However, these data sets, collected several years ago, were not designed to examine the reliability and validity of the DSM-5 SUD diagnosis. Field trials using standard methodology to minimize information variance are needed to provide information on DSM-5 SUD reliability that can be directly compared with DSM-IV, as well as studies on the antecedent, concurrent, and predictive validity of DSM-5 SUDs relative to DSM-IV dependence. The amount of data available to address the topics discussed above varied, and new studies will be needed for some of the more specific issues. However, the present recommendations for DSM-5 SUDs represent the results of a lengthy and intensive process aimed at identifying problems in DSM-IV and resolving them through changes in DSM-5.

References

American Psychiatric Association: Diagnostic and Statistical Manual of Mental Disorders, 4th Edition. Washington, DC, American Psychiatric Association, 1994

American Psychiatric Association: Diagnostic and Statistical Manual of Mental Disorders, 5th Edition. Washington, DC, American Psychiatric Association, 2013

Benowitz NL: Nicotine addiction. N Engl J Med 362(24):2295–2303, 2010

Budney AJ, Hughes JR: The cannabis withdrawal syndrome. Curr Opin Psychiatry 19(3):233–238, 2006

Casey M, Adamson G, Shevlin M, et al: The role of craving in AUDs: dimensionality and differential functioning in the DSM-5. Drug Alcohol Depend 125(1–2):75–80, 2012

Colgrove J, Bayer R, Bachynski KE: Nowhere left to hide? The banishment of smoking from public spaces. N Engl J Med 364(25):2375–2377, 2011

Copersino ML, Boyd SJ, Tashkin DP, et al: Cannabis withdrawal among non-treatment-seeking adult cannabis users. Am J Addict 15(1):8–14, 2006

Denis C, Fatseas M, Auriacombe M: Analyses related to the development of DSM-5 criteria for substance use related disorders: 3. An assessment of pathological gambling criteria. Drug Alcohol Depend 122(1–2):22–27, 2012

Grant BF, Harford TC, Muthen BO, et al: DSM-IV alcohol dependence and abuse: further evidence of validity in the general population. Drug Alcohol Depend 86(2–3):154–166, 2007

Guerri C, Bazinet A, Riley EP: Foetal alcohol spectrum disorders and alterations in brain and behaviour. Alcohol Alcohol 44(2):108–114, 2009

Hasin D, Paykin A, Endicott J, et al: The validity of DSM-IV alcohol abuse: drunk drivers versus all others. J Stud Alcohol 60(6):746–755, 1999

Hasin D, Hatzenbuehler ML, Keyes K, et al: Substance use disorders: Diagnostic and Statistical Manual of Mental Disorders, fourth edition (DSM-IV) and International Classification of Diseases, tenth edition (ICD-10). Addiction 101 (suppl 1):59–75, 2006

Hasin DS, Fenton MC, Beseler C, et al: Analyses related to the development of DSM-5 criteria for substance use related disorders: 2. Proposed DSM-5 criteria for alcohol, cannabis, cocaine and heroin disorders in 663 substance abuse patients. Drug Alcohol Depend 122(1–2):28–37, 2012

Hubbard R, Simpson D, Woody G: Treatment research: accomplishments and challenges. J Drug Issues 39:153–166, 2009

Hughes JR, Helzer JE, Lindberg SA: Prevalence of DSM/ICD-defined nicotine dependence. Drug Alcohol Depend 85(2):91–102, 2006

Juliano LM, Evatt DP, Richards BD, et al: Characterization of individuals seeking treatment for caffeine dependence. Psychol Addict Behav 26(4):948–954, 2012

Kessler RC, Hwang I, LaBrie R, et al: DSM-IV pathological gambling in the National Comorbidity Survey Replication. Psychol Med 38(9):1351–1360, 2008

Krueger RF, Nichol PE, Hicks BM, et al: Using latent trait modeling to conceptualize an alcohol problems continuum. Psychol Assess 16(2):107–119, 2004

National Institute on Alcohol Abuse and Alcoholism: Consensus statement on recognizing alcohol-related neurodevelopmental disorder (ARND) in primary health care of children. Bethesda, MD, National Institutes of Health, 2011. Available at: http://www.niaaa.nih.gov/sites/default/files/ARNDConferenceConsensusStatement Booklet_Complete.pdf. Accessed November 12, 2013.

Pollock NK, Martin CS: Diagnostic orphans: adolescents with alcohol symptom who do not qualify for DSM-IV abuse or dependence diagnoses. Am J Psychiatry 156(6):897–901, 1999

Saunders JB, Schuckit MA (eds): Diagnostic Issues in Substance Use Disorders: Refining the Research Agenda. Addiction 101 (suppl 1):1–173, 2006

Schuckit MA, Danko GP, Raimo EB, et al: A preliminary evaluation of the potential usefulness of the diagnoses of polysubstance dependence. J Stud Alcohol 62(1):54–61, 2001

Shmulewitz D, Wall MM, Aharonovich E, et al: Validity of proposed DSM-5 diagnostic criteria for nicotine use disorder: results from 734 Israeli lifetime smokers. Psychol Med 43(10):2179–2190, 2013

Tiffany ST, Friedman L, Greenfield SF, et al: Beyond drug use: a systematic consideration of other outcomes in evaluations of treatments for substance use disorders. Addiction 107(4):709–718, 2012

Urbina I: Addiction diagnoses may rise under guideline changes. The New York Times, May 11, 2012, p A11. Available at: http://www.nytimes.com/2012/05/12/us/dsm-revisions-may-sharply-increase-addiction-diagnoses.html?_r=2. Accessed November 12, 2013.

World Health Organization: The ICD-10 Classification of Mental and Behavioural Disorders: Diagnostic Criteria for Research. Geneva, Switzerland, World Health Organization, 1993

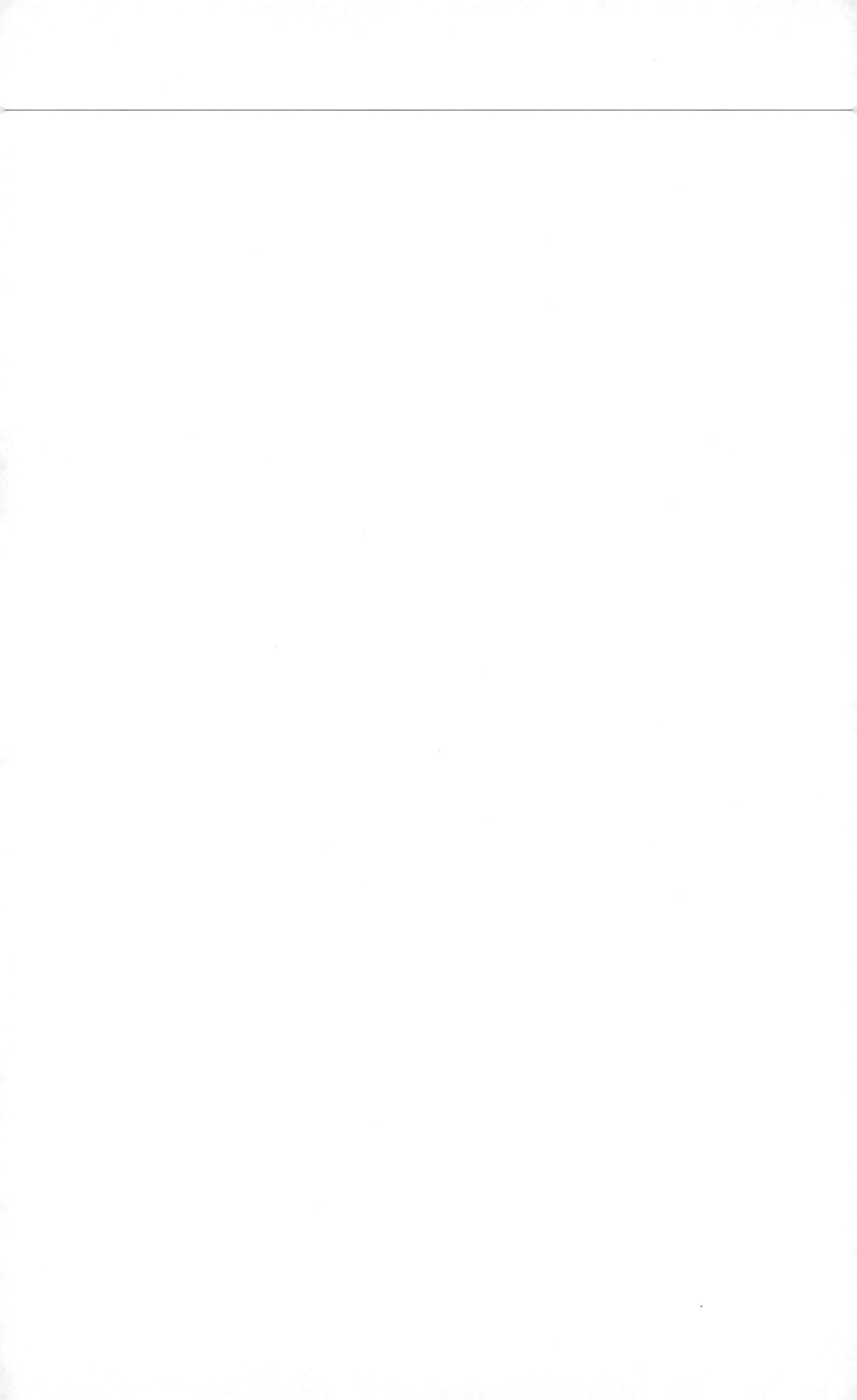

PART II

Substance-Related Disorders

CHAPTER 2

Alcohol

Conundrums of Co-occurring Disorders

Faye Chao, M.D.

ALCOHOL is one of the first psychoactive substances used by humans, with evidence of beer jugs dating back to 10,000 B.C. and wine first appearing in Egyptian pictographs by 4000 B.C. In modern times, alcohol is nearly ubiquitous; its presence can be noted on television, in film, on billboards, and in magazines. It is available for purchase not only in liquor stores but also in supermarkets, convenience stores, gas stations, and drive-throughs as well as on trains, planes, and boats. Given this wide accessibility, it is no surprise that in the United States, lifetime exposure is estimated to be as high as 86% (Substance Abuse and Mental Health Services Administration 2011). Despite this high rate of exposure, most people do not go on to develop an alcohol use disorder (Box 2–1). The National Epidemiologic Survey on Alcohol and Related Conditions estimated that lifetime prevalence for alcohol abuse was 17.8% and for alcohol dependence was 12.5%, with a total lifetime prevalence of 30.3% for any alcohol use disorder (Hasin et al. 2007).

Box 2–1. DSM-5 Criteria for Alcohol Use Disorder

A. A problematic pattern of alcohol use leading to clinically significant impairment or distress, as manifested by at least two of the following, occurring within a 12-month period:

1. Alcohol is often taken in larger amounts or over a longer period than was intended.
2. There is a persistent desire or unsuccessful efforts to cut down or control alcohol use.
3. A great deal of time is spent in activities necessary to obtain alcohol, use alcohol, or recover from its effects.
4. Craving, or a strong desire or urge to use alcohol.
5. Recurrent alcohol use resulting in a failure to fulfill major role obligations at work, school, or home.
6. Continued alcohol use despite having persistent or recurrent social or interpersonal problems caused or exacerbated by the effects of alcohol.
7. Important social, occupational, or recreational activities are given up or reduced because of alcohol use.
8. Recurrent alcohol use in situations in which it is physically hazardous.
9. Alcohol use is continued despite knowledge of having a persistent or recurrent physical or psychological problem that is likely to have been caused or exacerbated by alcohol.
10. Tolerance, as defined by either of the following:
    a. A need for markedly increased amounts of alcohol to achieve intoxication or desired effect.
    b. A markedly diminished effect with continued use of the same amount of alcohol.
11. Withdrawal, as manifested by either of the following:
    a. The characteristic withdrawal syndrome for alcohol (refer to Criteria A and B of the criteria set for alcohol withdrawal, DSM-5 pp. 499–500).
    b. Alcohol (or a closely related substance, such as a benzodiazepine) is taken to relieve or avoid withdrawal symptoms.

Specify if:

In early remission: After full criteria for alcohol use disorder were previously met, none of the criteria for alcohol use disorder have been met for at least 3 months but for less than 12 months (with the exception that Criterion A4, "Craving, or a strong desire or urge to use alcohol," may be met).

In sustained remission: After full criteria for alcohol use disorder were previously met, none of the criteria for alcohol use disorder have been met at any time during a period of 12 months or longer (with the exception that Criterion A4, "Craving, or a strong desire or urge to use alcohol," may be met).

Specify if:

In a controlled environment: This additional specifier is used if the individual is in an environment where access to alcohol is restricted.

Code based on current severity: Note for ICD-10-CM codes: If an alcohol intoxication, alcohol withdrawal, or another alcohol-induced mental disorder is also present, do not use the codes below for alcohol use disorder. Instead, the comorbid alcohol use disorder is indicated in the 4th character of the alcohol-induced disorder code (see the coding note for alcohol intoxication, alcohol withdrawal, or a specific alcohol-induced mental disorder). For example, if there is comorbid alcohol intoxication and alcohol use disorder, only the alcohol intoxication code is given, with the 4th character indicating whether the comorbid alcohol use disorder is mild, moderate, or severe: F10.129 for mild alcohol use disorder with alcohol intoxication or F10.229 for a moderate or severe alcohol use disorder with alcohol intoxication.

Specify current severity:

305.00 (F10.10) Mild: Presence of 2–3 symptoms.
303.90 (F10.20) Moderate: Presence of 4–5 symptoms.
303.90 (F10.20) Severe: Presence of 6 or more symptoms.

Source. Reprinted from the *Diagnostic and Statistical Manual of Mental Disorders,* 5th Edition, Washington, DC, American Psychiatric Association, 2013. Used with permission. Copyright © 2013 American Psychiatric Association.

Alcohol use disorder also carries significant morbidity and mortality. Chronic alcohol use has deleterious effects on many organ systems, including gastrointestinal, central nervous, and cardiovascular systems. Alcohol can be fatal in both intoxication (respiratory depression, aspiration) and withdrawal (delirium tremens) and can lead to disinhibition and lethal risk-taking behavior while intoxicated (motor vehicle accidents, falls, accidental discharge of firearms, etc.) (Boxes 2–2 and 2–3). Despite the impact of alcohol use disorder, access to treatment is limited, with one study finding that only 24.1% of patients who meet criteria for alcohol dependence ever receive treatment for this disorder (Hasin et al. 2007). Treatment usually employs a number of different modalities, including group therapy, counseling, individual psychotherapy, medication management, and peer-led groups, and patients may require several treatment episodes before achieving sobriety. The following case highlights some of the treatment settings and strategies available to patients struggling with alcohol use disorder.

Box 2–2. DSM-5 Criteria for Alcohol Intoxication

A. Recent ingestion of alcohol.
B. Clinically significant problematic behavioral or psychological changes (e.g., inappropriate sexual or aggressive behavior, mood lability, impaired judgment) that developed during, or shortly after, alcohol ingestion.
C. One (or more) of the following signs or symptoms developing during, or shortly after, alcohol use:
   1. Slurred speech.
   2. Incoordination.
   3. Unsteady gait.
   4. Nystagmus.
   5. Impairment in attention or memory.
   6. Stupor or coma.
D. The signs or symptoms are not attributable to another medical condition and are not better explained by another mental disorder, including intoxication with another substance.

Coding note: The ICD-9-CM code is **303.00.** The ICD-10-CM code depends on whether there is a comorbid alcohol use disorder. If a mild alcohol use disorder is comorbid, the ICD-10-CM code is **F10.129,** and if a moderate or severe alcohol use disorder is comorbid, the ICD-10-CM code is **F10.229.** If there is no comorbid alcohol use disorder, then the ICD-10-CM code is **F10.929.**

Source. Reprinted from the *Diagnostic and Statistical Manual of Mental Disorders,* 5th Edition, Washington, DC, American Psychiatric Association, 2013. Used with permission. Copyright © 2013 American Psychiatric Association.

Box 2–3. DSM-5 Criteria for Alcohol Withdrawal

A. Cessation of (or reduction in) alcohol use that has been heavy and prolonged.
B. Two (or more) of the following, developing within several hours to a few days after the cessation of (or reduction in) alcohol use described in Criterion A:
   1. Autonomic hyperactivity (e.g., sweating or pulse rate greater than 100 bpm).
   2. Increased hand tremor.
   3. Insomnia.
   4. Nausea or vomiting.
   5. Transient visual, tactile, or auditory hallucinations or illusions.
   6. Psychomotor agitation.
   7. Anxiety.
   8. Generalized tonic-clonic seizures.

C. The signs or symptoms in Criterion B cause clinically significant distress or impairment in social, occupational, or other important areas of functioning.
D. The signs or symptoms are not attributable to another medical condition and are not better explained by another mental disorder, including intoxication or withdrawal from another substance.

Specify if:

With perceptual disturbances: This specifier applies in the rare instance when hallucinations (usually visual or tactile) occur with intact reality testing, or auditory, visual, or tactile illusions occur in the absence of a delirium.

Coding note: The ICD-9-CM code is **291.81.** The ICD-10-CM code for alcohol withdrawal without perceptual disturbances is **F10.239,** and the ICD-10-CM code for alcohol withdrawal with perceptual disturbances is **F10.232.** Note that the ICD-10-CM code indicates the comorbid presence of a moderate or severe alcohol use disorder, reflecting the fact that alcohol withdrawal can only occur in the presence of a moderate or severe alcohol use disorder. It is not permissible to code a comorbid mild alcohol use disorder with alcohol withdrawal.

Source. Reprinted from the *Diagnostic and Statistical Manual of Mental Disorders,* 5th Edition, Washington, DC, American Psychiatric Association, 2013. Used with permission. Copyright © 2013 American Psychiatric Association.

Clinical Case

Rebecca is a 34-year-old white woman who was admitted initially for detoxification from alcohol. She previously had been living with her boyfriend of 5 years, but her drinking had been a point of contention in their relationship for the past year, and he had finally ended the relationship and moved out. Unable to pay their rent on her own and having recently lost her job, she was forced to move back in with her parents, with whom she had not lived since she was a college sophomore. Her parents, alarmed at her drinking and the recent changes in her life, were able to convince her to start cutting down on her own. However, she experienced a seizure 3 weeks prior to presentation and was taken to the emergency department, where she had a negative head computed tomography (CT) scan and was sent home. She resumed drinking at her previous level for the next 3 weeks, until she consented to be brought to the hospital for admission to the inpatient detoxification unit. After completing an uneventful course of detoxification, she was transferred to the rehabilitation unit. This was her first inpatient detoxification and rehabilitation, although she had done an outpatient detoxification approximately 4 years earlier before going to stay in a sober living house for 3 months. While on the rehab unit, Rebecca participated in group therapy, 12-step meetings, and individual therapy with her counselor. Her counselor noted that she appeared very anxious and fidgety in sessions and would easily become tearful; other counselors reported that she was quiet in group and also felt that she appeared anxious. Rebecca was seen by the psychiatrist on the unit for a formal evaluation during which the following history was elicited.

Rebecca reported having her first drink at age 14 while at a party with her friends. She recalled nothing special about this first experience, neither particularly liking nor disliking alcohol, but she had continued to drink "socially" through high school, mostly on the weekends. In college her drinking started to escalate somewhat, and she would binge more heavily on the weekends and would drink occasionally during the week as well. She remembered her drinking as not being significantly more than that of her peer group during weekend parties but admitted that most of her friends did not drink during the week. She also recalled one instance when she was taken to the student health center after she had passed out during a party and her friends were unable to rouse her. Her schoolwork was not affected, however, and she graduated with honors. She then moved to the West Coast to work in communications at a public relations firm.

Rebecca stated that it was at this time that she noticed a significant increase in her drinking. Drinks after work with coworkers were a frequent occurrence during the week, and Rebecca attended happy hours at least 3 days a week in addition to drinking on the weekends with her friends. Her work was enjoyable but also stressful, and she found herself either using alcohol to "reward" herself when projects were completed or, more often, drinking to de-stress after a long day. Initially, she had been able to perform well at work and had advanced in the firm, but additional responsibilities brought additional stress, and her drinking increased steadily until she was drinking daily. From ages 24 to 30, she estimated that she drank a bottle of wine daily. Her work eventually suffered as a result—excessive sick days, missed deadlines, strained relationships with peers—and although she never drank on the job, she was ultimately fired for her poor performance. It was around this time that Rebecca first entered treatment for her alcohol use with the outpatient detoxification and her stay at a sober living house. After treatment she had been able to remain sober only for a few weeks at a time and had not accessed any formal treatment, although she did intermittently attend Alcoholics Anonymous (AA) meetings.

Rebecca noted that she had always struggled with intense anxiety. She had been told that she was an anxious child, and she remembered feeling the scrutiny of others and constantly worrying about saying and doing the "right" things. This intensified when she was in the fourth grade and her family moved to a new town; her anxiety over being "different" and the "new kid at school" made her awkward around her peers and a target for teasing. Her anxiety persisted into adulthood, and although she was able to form close friendships, she still felt overwhelmed by new social situations. Her anxiety was not isolated to social situations but also encompassed worrying about school, work, bills, and so on. She noted that she often would have difficulty sleeping because she was worrying about things that had happened during the day and making plans for the next day. She felt that her mother, whom she most resembled, also had a "nervous" temperament and was known in the family as a "worrier," although she had never been diagnosed with any formal psychiatric illness. With respect to other family history, Rebecca's sister had depression and was taking medication, and Rebecca's father and grandfather had both been alcoholics. Rebecca was open about the fact that she found alcohol very effective in quelling her anxiety and that she was concerned that the significant stressors she was facing (lack of employment and independent housing and her recent breakup) would trigger her to relapse.

Rebecca also reported frequent mood lability—at times she could feel "good…almost happy" but then very suddenly become tearful or angry—with fluctuations from day to day rather than sustained periods of mood change. She felt that most of the time her mood tended toward a depressed state; she had had one brief observation period about 2 years previously when she reported worsened depressive symptoms and passive suicidal thoughts. She was discharged at that time with a diagnosis of major depressive disorder and had attended follow-up care with individual therapy and selective serotonin reuptake inhibitors (SSRIs) for a few months before discontinuing. Rebecca found therapy somewhat helpful but was unable to tolerate medication because she thought that it made her "too nervous." She denied periods of decreased need for sleep but did acknowledge difficulty getting to sleep because of anxiety. She had never had any psychotic symptoms (no hallucinations or grandiose delusions) or periods of euphoria. She did report sometimes spending more money than she had and neglecting to pay bills and loans in favor of buying presents for others; in a family meeting later in Rebecca's course her mother related that Rebecca had once taken a seemingly impulsive trip cross-country and had to have her parents buy a return ticket for her. While in the sober living house, her anxiety and depressed mood did not improve, and she continued to have frequent mood swings.

Rebecca was initially reluctant to start medication but ultimately decided that she had felt "not normal" for such a long time that "I'm willing to try anything." After a discussion of the risks, benefits, and alternatives to lamotrigine, she was started on a low dosage on the rehabilitation unit. She also was continued on buspirone 10 mg orally three times a day, which she had been prescribed by her primary care physician for anxiety; this was later discontinued because she had found it helpful only initially.

In individual sessions, Rebecca discussed further her fear that her anxiety would lead her to relapse. She admitted that after two drinks she sometimes felt that her worries were diminished and she was "almost normal." Because of this effect, she believed she was able to be more social and more functional, and she was fearful of giving this up. She was ambivalent about whether drinking helped her be more functional in other realms; she still believed that it had helped her manage work stress more effectively but admitted that when her drinking increased to daily, it eventually impaired her ability to work. Her therapist did not challenge her on these assertions and instead helped her highlight her reasons for wanting to quit drinking and consider what it might be like to lose these seemingly positive effects from alcohol. On further discussion, Rebecca realized that it had actually been quite some time since she had seen any of her friends with whom she was previously close and that in the latter stages of her alcohol use disorder she tended to be fairly isolative. She also worried about the effect that alcohol had had on her health and was quite rattled by her withdrawal seizure, which was one of the more direct precipitants that led her to seek treatment.

Rebecca did well over the course of her rehabilitation stay. She was an active participant in groups and worked in individual sessions on developing coping skills to manage anxiety. She attended AA groups while on the unit, but throughout her stay she questioned whether she could follow an abstinence-only approach long term. She did feel that early in her sobriety she would aim for abstinence. Her lamotrigine was titrated to a dosage of 50 mg orally twice daily, which she tolerated well. Rebecca reported a decrease in her overall level of anxiety and experienced somewhat improved mood with fewer mood swings. She was discharged after 28 days to continue treatment in an intensive outpatient program.

Discussion

A first step in planning a course of treatment may be helping the patient select a treatment setting. Fortunately for Rebecca, New York City has a number of options available. For patients requiring detoxification (i.e., patients using alcohol, benzodiazepines, or opioids), inpatient and outpatient detoxification services are available. For Rebecca, the main factor that drove her choice of inpatient detoxification was her alcohol withdrawal seizure, which occurs in about 3% of patients with alcohol dependence, thus necessitating closer monitoring and medical support services during detoxification. She then transitioned to inpatient rehabilitation because of her recent decline in functioning (lost job, boyfriend, housing) and suspicion of psychiatric comorbidity. Other treatment options available included an intensive outpatient program (could have been appropriate as well), long-term residential rehabilitation (likely too intensive), or outpatient treatment in a clinic setting (likely not intensive enough).

An important facet of this case was the fact that Rebecca had psychiatric symptoms that could have been related to her alcohol use or could have indicated a co-occurring psychiatric illness. Mood and anxiety disorders frequently co-occur with alcohol use disorders; results from the National Comorbidity Survey show 12-month prevalence rates of 12.3% and 29.1%, respectively, in alcohol abuse and 29.2% and 36.9% in alcohol dependence (Petrakis et al. 2002). In Rebecca's case, she was experiencing ongoing intense anxiety, mood swings (with mood more frequently depressed than elevated), and difficulty with sleep; she also had had periods in which she was spending more and engaging in impulsive behavior. She had had at least one major depressive episode in the past warranting a brief psychiatric observation. Determining whether her symptoms were substance induced or due to a co-occurring disorder required consideration of the time-course of the development of her symptoms and evaluation of her symptoms during previous periods of sobriety. Given that she described her childhood temperament as anxious, with intensification due to social upheaval in the fourth grade, it is clear that her anxiety preceded her substance use (which did not begin until age 15 and did not worsen to substance use disorder until her twenties). Depressive symptoms emerged in her college years and did not respond well to SSRIs. Rebecca's mood lability, which persisted even during a 3-month sobriety, her history of impulsive spending, and her cross-country trip made the team consider a diagnosis of bipolar II disorder. Lamotrigine helped stabilize her mood and diminished her anxiety enough for her to more fully participate in the treatment program available.

Although Rebecca did not choose to start a medication for the treatment of alcohol use disorder, there are three medication options available that are approved by the U.S. Food and Drug Administration (FDA). Of these medications, two—

acamprosate and naltrexone—are considered to have an "anticraving" effect, and the third—disulfiram—discourages patients from drinking by causing adverse reactions if patients drink while taking it. Disulfiram, which was the first of these medications available, acts to block the breakdown of acetaldehyde by aldehyde dehydrogenase; patients who drink while taking this medication experience nausea, flushing, palpitations, and headache. Disulfiram might be a good choice for patients who are motivated and have a supportive network to help with directly observed treatment. However, it does not reduce cravings, and patients can discontinue it and resume drinking within 2–3 days. Acamprosate, an *N*-methyl-D-aspartate modulator, and naltrexone, an opioid antagonist, both help to reduce cravings when taken daily. Although there is evidence supporting the efficacy of both, a large randomized controlled trial comparing the two showed superior efficacy for naltrexone (Anton et al. 2006).

Regarding Rebecca's attitude toward recovery, it is important to note that her therapist employed an empathic, patient-focused approach that is the spirit of motivational interviewing. Rather than confront her with reasons that she should be sober and the negatives that had come from her drinking, he allowed Rebecca to speak about some of the positive aspects she found from drinking and acknowledged that this would in some ways be a loss for her. Rebecca herself acknowledged that there were negative aspects to drinking, and her counselor worked with her to highlight these reasons for change and to enhance her motivation. This helped better engage her in treatment, created an empathic space for Rebecca in which to work on change, and prepared her for the next phase of treatment.

Key Points

- Alcohol use disorders are extremely common, with the majority of people having some lifetime exposure to alcohol and nearly a third of people meeting criteria for an alcohol use disorder at some point in their lives.
- Thoughtful selection of a treatment setting that matches the patient's needs at the time can be an important part of treatment planning.
- Determining whether psychiatric symptoms are substance induced or due to a co-occurring illness can be challenging, but ultimately, correctly identifying and treating co-occurring illness will aid patients in their recovery.
- Medications can be a useful adjunct to psychosocial treatments.

References

Anton RF, O'Malley SS, Ciraulo DA, et al: Combined pharmacotherapies and behavioral interventions for alcohol dependence. The COMBINE study: a randomized controlled trial. JAMA 295:2003–2017, 2006

Hasin DS, Stinson FS, Ogburn E, et al: Prevalence, correlates, disability, and comorbidity of DSM-IV alcohol abuse and dependence in the United States: results from the National Epidemiologic Survey on Alcohol and Related Conditions. Arch Gen Psychiatry 64:830–842, 2007

Petrakis IL, Gonzalez G, Rosenheck R, et al: Comorbidity of alcoholism and psychiatric disorders: an overview. Alcohol Research and Health 26:81–89, 2002. Available at: http://pubs.niaaa.nih.gov/publications/arh26-2/81-89.pdf. Accessed February 28, 2013.

Substance Abuse and Mental Health Services Administration: Results From the 2010 National Survey on Drug Use and Health: Summary of National Findings, NSDUH Series H-41, HHS Publication No (SMA) 11-4658. Rockville, MD, Substance Abuse and Mental Health Services Administration, 2011

Questions

2.1 Victoria presents to your office reporting depressed mood, anhedonia, poor sleep and appetite, low motivation, and difficulty concentrating for the past 3 months. She has been isolating more and finds that she is tearful sometimes for no reason. She also tells you that during the past 5 years she had been drinking a bottle of wine nightly, but 3 weeks ago she completed a detoxification and is currently still sober. What is the best next step?

A. Schedule the patient for a follow-up in 6 months because she should be sober for that period of time before you can accurately diagnose and treat a mood disorder.
B. Obtain a further history, particularly about her past periods of sobriety and any mood symptoms she might have experienced during those times, in order to establish a diagnosis before treatment.
C. Start her on low-dose benzodiazepines and taper slowly over the next month because she may be experiencing residual alcohol withdrawal symptoms.
D. Recommend that she attend Alcoholics Anonymous in her recovery program because sharing her story may improve her mood and help get her out of the house.

The correct answer is B.

Determining whether a patient's symptoms are substance induced or co-occurring is one of the more challenging aspects of working with patients with substance use disorders. One way in which we can start to differentiate is by establishing a time-course of the development of symptoms. This patient is early in her sobriety, but she may have had more extended periods of sobriety in the past, and the presence or absence of mood symptoms during these periods may aid you in diagnosis. You may also want to ask about time periods prior to the development of habitual substance use. Waiting for 6 months of sobriety after this visit may not be feasible because if she does have a co-occurring mood disorder, leaving it untreated for that period of time will likely jeopardize her sobriety. These symptoms are unlikely to be related only to withdrawal because the patient reports that they existed for several weeks prior to detoxification. Alcoholics Anonymous could be a useful adjunct to her recovery program, but again this does not address whether she has a mood disorder that could be treated at this time.

2.2 Michael is a 54-year-old man brought in by ambulance to the emergency department after having a witnessed generalized tonic-clonic seizure. He is accompanied by his wife, who provides history because the patient is initially somewhat confused in the postictal phase. She reports that Michael has been a heavy drinker for the past 15 years, drinking up to 1.5 pints of vodka daily, with his last drink about 72 hours prior to the seizure. She reports that he had another seizure in the past that was ultimately attributed to alcohol withdrawal. You note that he is tremulous and diaphoretic, with a blood pressure of 150/90 and a pulse in the 90s–100s. His head CT scan is negative. On reevaluation Michael's mental status has still not cleared—he is oriented only to name—and he is becoming belligerent, demanding to leave. Which of the following is the most appropriate next step?

A. Administer lorazepam 2 mg intramuscularly and admit to inpatient substance abuse rehabilitation unit.
B. Administer lorazepam 2 mg intramuscularly and admit to inpatient detoxification unit.
C. Administer lorazepam 2 mg intramuscularly and discharge him against medical advice.
D. Administer lorazepam 2 mg intramuscularly and admit to inpatient psychiatric unit.

The correct answer is B.

Michael has most likely had another alcohol withdrawal seizure and is currently exhibiting signs and symptoms of alcohol withdrawal. His confusion may be related either to being postictal or perhaps to developing delirium tremens (DTs). He requires immediate treatment of alcohol withdrawal (because a history of withdrawal seizures increases the risk for DTs, which carries a 20% mortality rate when untreated), and inpatient detoxification, rather than rehabilitation or psychiatric hospitalization, would be the appropriate treatment setting for him. Inpatient detoxification is for the most part (varies by state) a voluntary admission, and Michael is refusing treatment; however, his lack of orientation to date or place indicates that he lacks the capacity to make this medical decision, and he can be admitted for potentially life-saving treatment at this time despite his refusal.

2.3 John has a history of opioid use disorder that is now stabilized on methadone maintenance. He has been clean from heroin for 10 years but has increased his alcohol consumption and is now drinking a six-pack of beer daily. After completing an outpatient detoxification, he is now attending an intensive outpatient program to focus on his recovery from alcohol. He comes to see you in your primary care office because he is interested in medication to help him stop drinking. He says, "Methadone really helped me get back on my feet and kept me away from the heroin. I want to see if there's a medication that can help me for my drinking problem." Which of the following could be a useful adjunct to his regimen?

A. Naltrexone.
B. Disulfiram.
C. Lorazepam.
D. Acamprosate.
E. B and D.
F. A, B, and D.
G. All of the above.

The correct answer is E.

Disulfiram, acamprosate, and naltrexone are the only FDA-approved medications for the ongoing treatment of alcohol use disorders. Lorazepam, although useful in acute detoxification, has not shown any benefit as a "maintenance" medication in the way that methadone has for opioid use disorder. Because John is on methadone, naltrexone (an opioid antagonist) would not be an option for him, which leaves disulfiram and acamprosate.

CHAPTER 3

Caffeine

The Ins and Outs of Caffeine

Gary P. Katzman, M.D.

CAFFEINE (1,3,7-trimethylxanthine) is the most commonly used mood-altering drug and most socially acceptable stimulant in the world. Caffeine is found in dozens of plants, the most widely consumed being coffee and tea. Other substantial sources of caffeine include caffeinated soft drinks, cocoa products, some medications, and, increasingly, energy drinks and preparations.

Roughly 90% of all adults in the world consume caffeine in their daily diet. In developed countries, with the exception of England and Ireland, coffee is preferred over tea. Tea is preferred over coffee in developing countries, particularly in Asia, although increased interest in tea's purported health benefits has recently led to a rise in tea consumption in the United States. Average coffee consumption in the United States is about two cups per day, approximately 280 mg of caffeine. People who consume four or more cups of coffee per day are considered to be heavy users. Coffee consumption is higher in men than women. Caffeinated soft drinks are another significant source of caffeine, particularly for children. These drinks have a wide range of caffeine content, from 50 mg to more than 500 mg per can or bottle (Howland and Rohsenow 2013).

Although there is increased awareness that caffeine is a potentially addictive substance that may need further regulation given the explosive rise in the use of energy drinks, there has also been increased interest in its potentially beneficial effects. Caffeine affects multiple organ systems, including the central nervous, cardiovascular, endocrine, and gastrointestinal systems. The body of data on the effects of caffeine is growing, but currently, there is insufficient evidence to promote or discourage its consumption in the daily diet.

Clinical Case

George is a 28-year-old single man with a history of generalized anxiety disorder, panic attacks with a frequency of two or three per year, obsessive-compulsive disorder well controlled with fluvoxamine and ongoing cognitive-behavior therapy, and some mild acid reflux. He has recently felt more anxious after being promoted at his job in a factory and putting in longer hours at work. He reported feeling more sluggish during the day, which he attributed to greater difficulty falling asleep and the antihistamine he had been using recently for sinus troubles.

George reported that he drinks two large cups of coffee in the morning and "a few more" throughout the day. During the past few months he had been drinking energy drinks daily, sometimes up to four per day, particularly in light of his recent increase in fatigue. His energy drink consumption tends to increase in the afternoon and before going out if he thinks it will be a late night. He and his friends also use caffeine to counteract the sedative effect of alcohol and have found that it allows them to drink more alcohol before feeling sedated or passing out. They have become fans of the increasingly popular combination of Red Bull and vodka. When George goes out and drinks alcohol, he often smokes a few cigarettes. He reported having tried marijuana and cocaine in the past but had not used either in the past 4 years.

George used to go to the gym regularly each morning before going to work but stopped with the advent of almost daily headaches. These headaches tend to last for about an hour and then subside.

Two weeks ago, on his fourth day of treatment with the antibiotic ciprofloxacin for an infectious sinusitis and 6 days after quitting cigarettes "cold turkey" on the advice of his ear, nose, and throat doctor, George was brought to the emergency department complaining of chest pain, diaphoresis, and difficulty breathing.

Discussion

Coffee is the leading dietary source of caffeine among adults in the United States, and soft drinks represent the largest source of caffeine for children. Tea consumption in the United States has been increasing, and over the past few decades caffeine consumption from soft drinks has dramatically increased, with 70% of all soft drinks containing caffeine, but the most dramatic change has been in the energy drink and product segment. It may be the tremendous variety in flavors offered by coffees, teas, and soft drinks that entices the consumer, but similar to the effects of alcohol, it is the desirable effects of the caffeine that make it the alluring Siren that it is.

Effects of Caffeine

Caffeine consumption leads to increased alertness, energy, and ability to concentrate, particularly when subjects are fatigued. Its main effects stem from its action as a potent antagonist at central and peripheral nervous system adenosine receptors. This leads to a net stimulating effect on excitatory neurotransmitters.

Studies have shown that caffeine in amounts as small as 30 mg or less can alter mood and affect behavior, and 100 mg of caffeine per day can lead to physical dependence and withdrawal symptoms on discontinuation. The mood-altering effects of caffeine depend on the amount of caffeine consumed, the individual's sensitivity to caffeine, and how rapidly the caffeine is metabolized. In noncaffeine or intermittent users, low doses of caffeine (20–200 mg) generally produce the desired effects of increased arousal and alertness and a sense of well-being. Among daily caffeine users, the predominant effect experienced with consumption of caffeine in the morning after overnight abstinence is suppression of low-grade withdrawal symptoms such as sleepiness and lethargy. Large amounts of caffeine, often greater than 500 mg, may produce negative mood effects. Although generally mild and brief, these effects include increased anxiety, nervousness, jitteriness, and upset stomach. The potential for negative effects is largely dependent on dose, sensitivity, and tolerance. Very high doses of caffeine can lead to caffeine intoxication, characterized by agitation, anxiety, tremors, tachycardia, diuresis, gastrointestinal upset, muscle twitching, insomnia, and symptoms that mimic mania such as pressured speech and racing thoughts, paranoia, and a decreased need for sleep (Box 3–1). There have been reports of fatalities at exceptionally high doses, typically of the order of 5–10 g. Most deaths were a result of arrhythmias (Heatherley 2011).

In addition to its effects on mood and energy, caffeine is strongly associated with enhanced athletic performance, both in endurance and in sprinting feats. The International Olympic Committee actually prohibits urinary caffeine concentrations greater than 12 mcg/mL, which is roughly the equivalent of three to six cups of coffee depending on factors that affect clearance.

The effects of caffeine emerge quickly because it is absorbed quite rapidly from the gastrointestinal tract, with a peak blood level achieved in less than 1 hour. Food slows but does not inhibit the absorption of caffeine. The half-life generally ranges from 2 to 7 hours, with an average of 5 hours. Those who metabolize caffeine more slowly may experience jitteriness that persists throughout the day, as well as sleep-onset and sleep-maintenance insomnias, even if caffeine is used only in the morning hours (Substance Abuse and Mental Health Services Administration, Center for Behavioral Health Statistics and Quality 2013).

Box 3–1. DSM-5 Criteria for Caffeine Intoxication **305.90 (F15.929)**

A. Recent consumption of caffeine (typically a high dose well in excess of 250 mg).
B. Five (or more) of the following signs or symptoms developing during, or shortly after, caffeine use:
   1. Restlessness.
   2. Nervousness.
   3. Excitement.
   4. Insomnia.
   5. Flushed face.
   6. Diuresis.
   7. Gastrointestinal disturbance.
   8. Muscle twitching.
   9. Rambling flow of thought and speech.
   10. Tachycardia or cardiac arrhythmia.
   11. Periods of inexhaustibility.
   12. Psychomotor agitation.
C. The signs or symptoms in Criterion B cause clinically significant distress or impairment in social, occupational, or other important areas of functioning.
D. The signs or symptoms are not attributable to another medical condition and are not better explained by another mental disorder, including intoxication with another substance.

Source. Reprinted from the *Diagnostic and Statistical Manual of Mental Disorders,* 5th Edition, Washington, DC, American Psychiatric Association, 2013. Used with permission. Copyright © 2013 American Psychiatric Association.

Metabolism occurs primarily in the liver by demethylation and oxidation by the cytochrome P450 1A2 (CYP1A2) enzyme. Genetic polymorphisms in the CYP1A2 pathway and substances that affect this enzyme's production may affect caffeine's half-life and the duration of its effects. Two of the metabolites, theophylline and theobromine, are also active stimulants.

There are a number of inducers and inhibitors of this particular enzyme that may affect the intensity and duration of the effects of caffeine. The selective serotonin reuptake inhibitor (SSRI) fluvoxamine, used predominantly for the treatment of obsessive-compulsive spectrum disorders because it was the first to receive U.S. Food and Drug Administration (FDA) approval for that indication, is a potent CYP450 1A2 inhibitor. The fluoroquinolone antibiotic ciprofloxacin (Cipro) also substantially inhibits CYP1A2. These two medications therefore can lead to clinically increased blood levels of caffeine. Although cigarettes are potent inducers of CYP1A2 activity, leading to more rapid metabolism of caffeine, abrupt cessation of cigarette use can be followed by a marked increase in sensitivity to the effects of caffeine because the body registers the change as a net increase in caffeine. As seen in the clinical case, George found himself in a perfect storm and in the hospital with elevated blood caffeine levels and a panic attack. Likely contributors included the net CYP1A2 inhibition after the initiation of ciprofloxacin and the abrupt discontinuation of cigarettes in the context of his continued maintenance on fluvoxamine for obsessive-compulsive disorder symptoms and his recent increase in caffeine, which was intended to combat the increased fatigue that was likely stemming from his infection, use of sedating antihistamines, and decreased physical activity (Substance Abuse and Mental Health Services Administration, Center for Behavioral Health Statistics and Quality 2013).

Assessment

Patients' reports of amount and frequency of substance use have been shown to be inaccurate representations of actual use. Further complicating the issue of obtaining an accurate use history, caffeine content varies greatly depending on size, beverage, and preparation. Although tea and soft drinks usually contain about one-half to one-third the amount of caffeine in a serving of coffee, this amount can vary greatly with the product and how it is prepared. Historically, colas were caffeinated and noncola sodas were not. Today, many noncola drinks such as root beer, orange soda, and cream soda contain caffeine in amounts similar to those in cola drinks. Some, but not all, coffee ice creams and yogurts contain a significant amount of caffeine. Most chocolate milk, cocoa, and milk chocolate candy contain small amounts of caffeine, and a serving of dark chocolate candy may contain about 30 mg of caffeine, reaching the threshold of noticeable effects. The clinical case description leaves us with a very poor understanding of George's actual caffeine use. A thorough assessment needs to include data on what he is using, including the different formulations and preparations, quantity and frequency of use, effects of the substance, consequences of use, motivation to change use, and trials at decreasing or stopping use.

Particular attention needs to be paid in any thorough assessment to the often neglected but commonly used medicinal, recreational, and food products that contain caffeine (see Tables 3–1, 3–2, and 3–3). Over-the-counter medicinal products such as NoDoz and Vivarin, used to combat somnolence, contain between 100 and 200 mg per tablet, whereas analgesics such as Anacin, Excedrin, and Midol contain 64–130 mg per dose. Energy strips and energy drinks also need to be considered, especially in light of their explosive increase in popularity. In particular, with young male patients such as George, physicians should ask their patients about their use of energy drinks.

Aside from important data being gathered, the assessment can be an important step in helping the patient reframe how caffeine-containing products are viewed. Many people see them as harmless and with few reasons for concern.

TABLE 3–1. Caffeine content in beverages

Beverage	Fluid ounces	Caffeine per fluid ounce (mg)	Total caffeine (mg)
24:7 Energy	16	10	160
5-Hour Energy	2	69	138
5150 Juice (concentrate)	32	500	16,000
7-Up	12	0	0
70 mg Energy mix (concentrate)	2.5	280	700
Arizona Iced Tea	20	1.9	38
Arizona Caution energy drink	16	12.5	200
Barq's Root Beer	12	1.9	23
Chocolate milk	8	0.6	5
Coca-Cola Classic	12	2.8	34
Coffee (brewed)	8	13.4	108
Coffee (decaf, brewed)	8	0.7	6
Coffee (drip)	8	18.1	145
Dr Pepper	12	3.4	41
McDonald's large coffee	16	9.1	145
Monster energy drink	16	10	160
Mountain Dew	12	4.5	54
Pepsi-Cola	12	3.2	38
Pure KWK energy drink	12	25	300
Red Bull	8.46	9.5	80
Snapple Tea	16	2.6	42
Starbucks grande coffee	16	20.6	330
Sunkist orange soda	12	3.4	41
Tea (brewed)	8	5.9	47
Tea (brewed, imported)	8	7.5	60
Tea (green)	8	3.1	25
Venom Death Adder	16	10	160
Vitamin Energy Attention	20	4.3	87
Whoop Ass energy drink	16	6.2	100
Xtreme Shock energy drink	12	16.7	200
Yerba Mate tea	8	10.6	85

TABLE 3–2. Caffeine content in foods

Product	Total caffeine (mg)
Häagen-Dazs coffee ice cream	48 per 8 oz cup
Starbucks coffee ice cream	60 per 8 oz cup
Ben and Jerry's coffee ice cream	70 per 8 oz cup
Bang!! caffeinated ice cream	250 per 8 oz cup
Clif energy bar, Peanut Toffee Buzz	50 per bar
Alien Energy jerky	110 per packet
Baking chocolate (squares)	23 per 29 g square
Hershey's milk chocolate bars	9 per 1.55 oz bar
Hershey's Special Dark bars	18 per 1.45 oz bar
Hershey's Kiss	1 per Kiss
Stay Puft caffeinated marshmallows	100 per marshmallow
Caffeinated maple bacon lollipop	80 per lollipop
Energy Sheets	50 per sheet
AMP energy gum	40 per piece
Jolt gum	45 per piece
Revive energy mint	102 per mint

Caffeinated Energy Drinks and Energy Strips

Energy drinks first made their debut in the United States as recently as 1997. In 2010, roughly 6 billion energy drinks were sold in the United States, with subsequent logarithmic growth. The majority of energy drink consumers are men between the ages of 18 and 24. Some studies suggest that up to 50% of young adults regularly consume these products (Reissig et al. 2009). Recently, while in my local supermarket, I noticed a display in the front of one of the aisles near the cash register. There were seven different brands of energy drinks and multiple varieties in some of the brands. The size of the containers ranged from 8 to 20 oz. Clearly, there is a battle for market share in this rapidly growing beverage segment. There are more than 500 different energy drinks available in North America, 25 different ones made under the Monster Energy drink label alone, some with very catchy names. Gone is the era of subtlety, when those who wished to be pepped up ordered a Dr Pepper. Today, one can order an Xtreme Shock Energy Drink or a Venom Death Adder, and the expression "opening a can of Whoop Ass" may be taken literally with use of the Whoop Ass Energy Drink. The energy drink Cocaine has recently changed its name but is still traded on eBay.

TABLE 3–3. Caffeine content in medications

Product	Total caffeine (mg)
Anacin	32 per tablet
Excedrin	65 per pill
Alka-Seltzer Wake-up Call	65 per pill
NoDoz	100 per pill
NoDoz Maximum Strength	200 per pill
Vivarin	200 per pill
Hydroxycut Hardcore	100 per capsule
Pharmacia Latex Aktiebolaget condoms	In lubricant
Turbo Snort energy nasal spray	1 per spray
Spot On energy patch	20 per transdermal patch

Most energy drinks contain roughly 10 mg caffeine per ounce. Given the size of these containers, consumers are ingesting roughly 160–240 mg of caffeine per can. Coca-Cola has 35 mg of caffeine in its 12 oz can, whereas Monster Energy drink contains 120 mg and 5-Hour Energy shots (2 oz drinks sold in supermarkets and convenience stores) contain between 157 and 206 mg depending on the variety. Energy strips typically contain roughly 100 mg caffeine per two-strip serving (Sepkowitz 2013). The market leader in this product segment, cofounded by basketball star LeBron James, is aggressively marketing its strips as convenient, portable, and less expensive alternatives to other caffeinated products. Estimated sales projections predict energy strips will become a billion-dollar segment in 3–5 years.

Given that most energy drinks also contain substances that are considered herbal or "natural," they fall under guidelines for dietary supplements and are not obligated to disclose their caffeine content, although many do. Some of these natural additives are active compounds such as taurine and guarana, a stimulant similar to caffeine, as well as sugars.

Caffeine Mixed With Alcohol

As many as 50% of college students report mixing energy drinks with alcohol. Vodka mixed with Red Bull energy drink—also known as vodka Red Bull, VARB, VRB, VKRB, Red Bull and vodka, RBV, Speedball, or Vod-Bomb—has become a popular cocktail among those 18–30 years old. The number of nicknames, acronyms, and aliases certainly speaks to its popularity. The ratio of Red Bull to vodka is typically 3:1 (Howland and Rohsenow 2013). There are also now commercially available premixed beverages containing varying amounts of caffeine and alcohol. Many consumers of this mixture simply drink the caffeine and alcohol separately but in the same drinking period.

Users of this combination do so to decrease the sedative effect of alcohol, allowing them to consume more alcohol. Caffeine may mask the effects of alcohol and can reduce perception of alcohol intoxication. In some studies, although caffeine did enhance reaction times in those who were using alcohol, when compared with an alcohol-only group, error rates did not differ. The false sense of safety one may achieve with this beverage mixture may actually lead to increased rates of morbidity and mortality. In a study of students from 10 U.S. universities, students who used this mixture were twice as likely to be exposed to or to commit a sexual assault. They were also twice as likely to be involved in a motor vehicle accident (Howland and Rohsenow 2013).

In 2010, under increasing legal and government pressures, the most popular alcohol-energy drink manufacturer reformulated its product, removing the stimulants. In 2012 the FDA declared the combination of caffeine and alcohol unsafe.

Other Caffeinated Products

Aside from more traditional sources, we might continue to see the addition of caffeine into a wider array of products. For example, if sex is not stimulating enough, a Swedish company, Pharmacia Latex Aktiebolaget, has developed a condom that contains caffeine in the lubricant. People with a more childlike sensibility may try Stay Puft caffeinated marshmallows, with 100 mg caffeine in each marshmallow (perhaps in combination with a favorite caffeine-free diet soda, of course). If one is short on time or eggs, there is always breakfast consisting of a caffeinated maple bacon lollipop, containing 80 mg of caffeine.

Psychiatric and Medical Sequelae of Caffeine Use

Among all the substances considered to have addiction potential, caffeine has been one of the most investigated for both its negative and its beneficial effects. Although there is a clear relationship between caffeine and neuropsychiatric sequelae, many of the studies that have explored the risks and benefits to other organ systems have actually looked at coffee and tea, which contain multiple compounds that have pharmacological effects. Most of these compounds are antioxidants.

More than 20,000 U.S. emergency department visits in 2011 were related to the use of energy drinks, nearly double the amount recorded in 2007 (see Figure 3–1). Heavy caffeine use is comorbid with other addictive substances, including tobacco and alcohol. Caffeinated drinks often involve the use of additive substances, some of which may have negative effects on health. Products such as cream, nondairy creamers, milk, sugar, and other additives often found in energy drinks, such as taurine, creatine, and carnitine, may have varying effects on endocrine and cardiovascular health (Sepkowitz 2013).

Anxiety

I have had many conversations with patients who swear that caffeine does not lead to or exacerbate their anxiety. Some have been willing to taper their caffeinated beverage and switch to a high-quality decaffeinated variety, understanding that decaffeinated coffee does indeed have some caffeine. I have received some enthusiastic testimonials asserting a reduction in anxiety following the taper and a rebound in anxiety when regular caffeinated beverages are reintroduced. Studies have shown that high doses of caffeine, typically 200 mg or more, increase self-report of anxiety and may precipitate panic attacks in the general population. Individuals with anxiety disorders are particularly sensitive to the effects of caffeine, which may be elicited at lower doses. Some highly anxious people will naturally avoid caffeine use; however, many are not aware of the relationship between caffeine and anxiety, and many fail to recognize the role that caffeine plays in their anxiety. Thousands of emergency department visits each year are due to anxiety or panic attacks, many precipitated or exacerbated by the use of stimulants, including caffeine.

Sleep

As a neuronal excitatory substance, caffeine generally negatively affects sleep. Consumption before bedtime or in the latter part of the day results in increased sleep latency, decreased total sleep time, and decreased slow wave deep sleep, with more frequent awakenings. Habituated users of caffeine typically are less susceptible to the effects of caffeine on sleep. Although disruptions in sleep may be experienced with one or even less than one cup of coffee in the morning, disruption in sleep is generally related to the dose of caffeine and the time of administration. The same modifying factors that may alter caffeine's rate of metabolism, as discussed earlier, will have similar effects on sleep disruption (Substance Abuse and Mental Health Services Administration, Center for Behavioral Health Statistics and Quality 2013).

Headache

Caffeine is modestly effective in relieving tension-type and migraine headaches. It increases analgesic effects by up to 40%. It also facilitates more rapid absorption of the analgesic. Usually, greater than 65 mg of caffeine is necessary to demonstrate analgesic effects. There are many over-the-counter as well as prescription medications available containing varying doses of caffeine. Chronic use of these medications may lead to rebound headaches due to interdose withdrawal from the caffeine (Reissig et al. 2009).

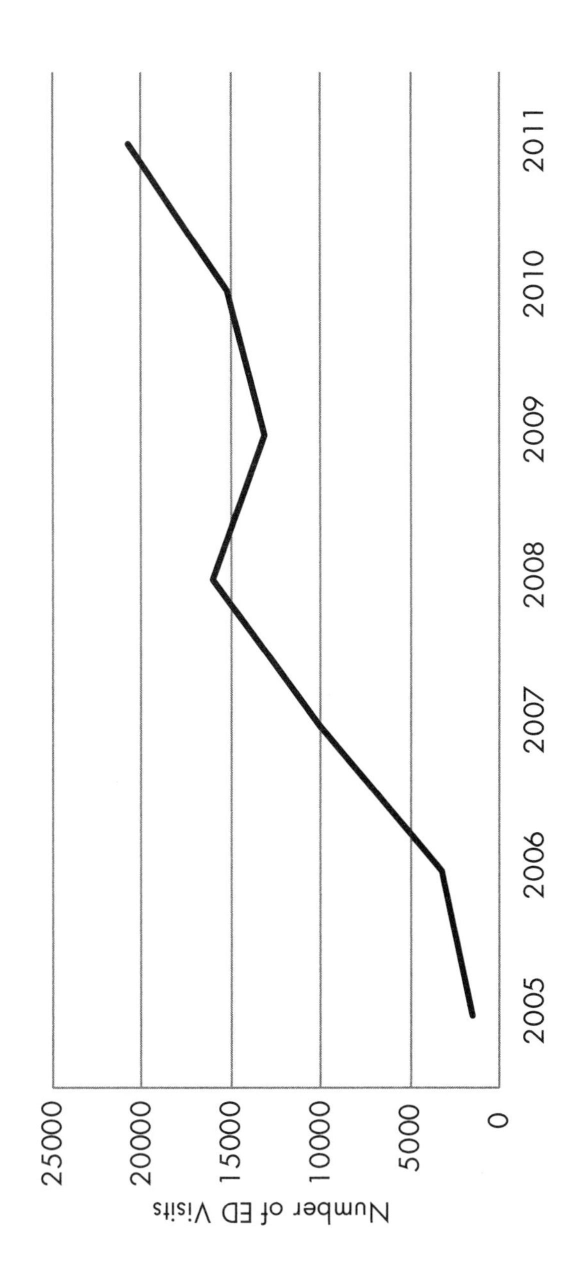

FIGURE 3–1. Energy drink–related emergency department (ED) visits by year, 2005–2011.
Source. Substance Abuse and Mental Health Services Administration, Center for Behavioral Health Statistics and Quality 2013.

Parkinson's and Alzheimer's Diseases

Coffee and tea are associated with a reduced risk of Parkinson's disease. In women who are taking postmenopausal hormone replacement therapy, caffeine consumption might actually increase the risk for Parkinson's disease. These data suggest a possible interaction between coffee and hormone use.

Between 2009 and 2012, a few studies in both mice and humans suggested a small protective effect against Alzheimer's disease. The dose of caffeine needed to achieve some effect was between three and five cups of coffee per day.

Gastrointestinal Effects

Caffeine leads to a rapid rise in gastric acid secretion. Through its action on smooth muscle, it relaxes the upper-esophageal sphincter, allowing gastric contents to flow up into the esophagus. These factors contribute to an increased incidence of heartburn and gastroesophageal reflux disease.

A large U.S. study demonstrated a strong inverse dose-dependent relationship between coffee and alcoholic cirrhosis. A lower rate of disease progression in patients with advanced hepatitis C infection was also noted.

Cardiovascular and Endocrine Effects

Low to moderate coffee consumption may protect against myocardial infarction. Particularly in heavy caffeine users, intake may increase the risk for arrhythmias; however, these events may occur at lower caffeine doses in susceptible individuals. These arrhythmias sometimes lead to outpatient or emergency department visits.

Caffeine consumption is associated with a reduced risk of diabetes. A few prospective, long-term studies have demonstrated that consumption of coffee or tea is correlated with improved insulin sensitivity and better control of postprandial glycemia in patients with diabetes. However, a recent study suggests a dose-dependent decrease in insulin sensitivity in both men and women. It is likely that some of the other compounds in coffee and tea may be responsible for these benefits because decaffeinated coffee is also associated with a lower risk of type 2 diabetes and lower HbA1C concentrations.

Cancer

Research is inconsistent on the effects of coffee and tea in various cancers, despite the assumption that the numerous antioxidants found within them might be protective.

Miscellaneous Illnesses and Caffeine

Caffeine has been correlated with a reduction in the risk for gout. Coffee, particularly with heavy consumption, may be associated with lower bone mineral density, whereas tea consumption has been associated with a higher bone mineral density. Coffee might lead to an increased risk for fractures, especially in calcium-deficient women, whereas tea has not been shown to confer a decreased fracture risk. It is thought that the higher flavonoids in tea might be responsible for the effect of greater bone mineral density. There are no data to support the old wives' tale that coffee stunts growth in children. Caffeine has mild diuretic properties, perhaps less robust than previously thought, as suggested by recent studies.

Caffeine-Related Disorders

Like most substances that have the potential for addiction, caffeine acts as a self-reinforcer. Its very use increases the likelihood that it will again be consumed, independent of its effects, whether desirable or not. Although there are case studies demonstrating tolerance to caffeine, clinical indicators of frank addiction to caffeine have not been clearly demonstrated, and there is a debate whether tolerance even develops. Although DSM-5 (American Psychiatric Association 2013) provides criteria for caffeine intoxication and caffeine withdrawal as valid, independent disorders, it does not include caffeine use disorder as a diagnosis.

Caffeine Withdrawal

After sudden cessation of caffeine, many people will experience a range of unpleasant signs and symptoms, commonly referred to as caffeine withdrawal (Box 3–2). Up to 50% of those with abrupt cessation of caffeine may experience caffeine withdrawal. These signs and symptoms typically emerge 12–24 hours after terminating caffeine intake, although onset as late as 36 hours has been documented. The duration of withdrawal for most people is roughly 1 day, lasting up to 1 week in some. Given the relatively short half-life of caffeine, most chronic users of caffeine actually experience daily morning withdrawal that is relieved by their morning coffee or tea. The most commonly described withdrawal symptom is headache, often gradual in onset and diffuse in location, usually mild but sometimes throbbing and severe. Other common features include fatigue, drowsiness, psychomotor retardation, deceased concentration, irritability, anxiety, and decreased mood. Some people even experience flu-like symptoms (Heatherley 2011).

Box 3–2. DSM-5 Criteria for Caffeine Withdrawal **292.0 (F15.93)**

A. Prolonged daily use of caffeine.
B. Abrupt cessation of or reduction in caffeine use, followed within 24 hours by three (or more) of the following signs or symptoms:
   1. Headache.
   2. Marked fatigue or drowsiness.
   3. Dysphoric mood, depressed mood, or irritability.
   4. Difficulty concentrating.
   5. Flu-like symptoms (nausea, vomiting, or muscle pain/stiffness).
C. The signs or symptoms in Criterion B cause clinically significant distress or impairment in social, occupational, or other important areas of functioning.
D. The signs or symptoms are not associated with the physiological effects of another medical condition (e.g., migraine, viral illness) and are not better explained by another mental disorder, including intoxication or withdrawal from another substance.

Source. Reprinted from the *Diagnostic and Statistical Manual of Mental Disorders,* 5th Edition, Washington, DC, American Psychiatric Association, 2013. Used with permission. Copyright © 2013 American Psychiatric Association.

Treatment

The first step in treating caffeine overuse is for patients to learn about the potential consequences of use and to understand the interaction between their use and outcomes. One way to do this is by doing a functional analysis. A functional analysis is an assessment of the chain of events that precede and follow the use of a substance. Helping caffeine users to understand the antecedents, or the potential triggers, and the consequences of their use can be an integral part of changing their use patterns.

To facilitate abstinence while reducing the chance of withdrawal symptoms, it is recommended that caffeine intake be gradually reduced over the course of 1 week. Not everyone will experience withdrawal symptoms. This is somewhat dependent on length of use and amount, and on polymorphisms of the adenosine receptor *A2A* gene. This is consistent with the reduction in caffeine intake by individuals homozygous for an adenosine receptor *A2A* gene variant. For many caffeine users, there is a lack of withdrawal symptoms on abrupt discontinuation. For most of those who do have withdrawal symptoms, the discomfort tends to be mild. Therefore, unplanned, abrupt discontinuation (e.g., from an emergency procedure) is not typically treated with caffeine replacement as are many other substances with a withdrawal profile.

Although there are treatment facilities that report helping patients detoxify from caffeine, they are rarely used (Heatherley 2011).

Key Points

- Many people are unaware of the health risks of caffeine and the wide range of users' susceptibility to its effects.
- There are a number of cytochrome P450 interactions that can affect the rate of metabolism and the effects of caffeine.
- There is a trend toward increased caffeine consumption, primarily through the use of energy drinks.
- There are potentially dangerous interactions between caffeine and alcohol, which is becoming an increasingly popular combination.

References

American Psychiatric Association: Diagnostic and Statistical Manual of Mental Disorders, 5th Edition. Washington, DC, American Psychiatric Association, 2013

Heatherley SV: Caffeine withdrawal, sleepiness, and driving performance: what does the research really tell us? Nutr Neurosci 14:89–95, 2011

Howland J, Rohsenow DJ: Risk of energy drinks mixed with alcohol. JAMA 309:245–246, 2013

Reissig CJ, Strain EC, Griffiths RR: Caffeinated energy drinks: a growing problem. Drug Alcohol Depend 99:1–10, 2009

Sepkowitz K: Energy drinks and caffeine: related adverse effects. JAMA 309:243–244, 2013

Substance Abuse and Mental Health Services Administration, Center for Behavioral Health Statistics and Quality: The DAWN Report: Update on Emergency Department Visits Involving Energy Drinks: A Continuing Public Health Concern. Rockville, MD, Substance Abuse and Mental Health Services Administration, 2013

Questions

3.1 The most likely users of energy drinks are

A. Males 18–24 years old.
B. Females 10–24 years old.
C. Males 35–50 years old.
D. Females 35–50 years old.

The correct answer is A.

Most consumers of energy drinks are men between the ages of 18 and 24. However, the use of energy drinks in older adults, regardless of gender, is increasing.

3.2 Cigarette smoking affects caffeine metabolism by being a potent ________ of the cytochrome P450 1A2 enzyme.

A. Substrate.
B. Inhibitor.
C. Inducer.
D. None of the above.

The correct answer is C.

Cigarette smoking leads to an increase in cytochrome P450 1A2 enzyme production. This results in a faster clearance of caffeine through an increase in its metabolism. Abrupt cessation of cigarette smoking will lead to a brisk rebound in caffeine blood levels.

3.3 The effects of caffeine are related to

A. Genetics.
B. Amount of use.
C. Interactions of other substances with the CYP450 system.
D. All of the above.

The correct answer is D.

The effects of caffeine are related to a complex array of factors, including genes, amount of use, and rate of metabolism by the cytochrome P450 1A2 enzyme system.

3.4 The combination of caffeine and alcohol

A. Decreases the rate of alcohol-related accidents by reducing sedation.
B. Increases the rate of sexual assaults.
C. Is illegal in most states.
D. Is decreasing in popularity.

The correct answer is B.

It has been shown that people who mix caffeine with alcohol are at increased risk for being exposed to or propagating a sexual assault.

3.5 The most commonly experienced symptom of caffeine withdrawal is

A. Nausea.
B. Tremor.
C. Tachycardia.
D. Headache.

The correct answer is D.

Headache is the most common side effect associated with caffeine withdrawal.

CHAPTER 4

Cannabis

A Natural Dilemma

TIMOTHY K. BRENNAN, M.D., M.P.H.
SAADIQ J. BEY, M.S.W., CASAC, ICADC

CANNABIS, otherwise known as marijuana, is a naturally occurring plant that is used around the world as a psychostimulant. There are innumerable historical and cultural examples of human beings using (and abusing) cannabis. Although some countries and several states in the United States have recently begun to reassess the legality of cannabis, these issues remain outside the scope of this chapter. Cannabis, like alcohol, tobacco, and other drugs, remains a potential individual and public health hazard.

Epidemiology of Cannabis Use

The cannabis plant is grown and cultivated in almost every country on Earth and is the most commonly used illegal drug (Kaminer 2008). According to the World Health Organization, up to 4% of the world's population between 15 and 64 years of age tried cannabis in 2004. Up to 42% of Americans over the age of 16 have tried cannabis at least once in their lives, and 9% would meet criteria for cannabis use disorder at some time in their lives (Box 4–1). National prevalence rates for active cannabis use remain around 9%. Prevalence is highest among younger Americans ages 18–25 (23%) and decreases as age increases: ages 26–34 (14%), ages 35–49 (7%), and ages above 50 (1%). Across all ages, cannabis use (not dependence or abuse) is higher among men and greater for blacks (10.6%) than whites (8.9%) or Hispanics (8.6%). Cannabis use is higher among divorced or separated adults and higher among those without a high school diploma compared with those with a college degree. Cannabis abuse and dependence develop within a mean of 2 years after the age of first use and do not show any racial or demographic risk factors. Patients who continually use cannabis are more likely to abuse other psychoactive substances than those who do not (Dutra et al. 2008): 90% of cannabis users use alcohol, 68% use nicotine, and 12% use cocaine. Cannabis users are more likely to have co-occurring psychiatric disease than people who do not use cannabis. The prevalence of cannabis use among patients with psychiatric disease is as follows (Conway et al. 2006):

- Schizophrenia, 31%
- Mania, 30%
- Dysthymia, 22%
- Hypomania, 21%
- Major depressive disorder, 16%
- Panic disorder with agoraphobia, 26%
- Generalized anxiety disorder, 19%

Box 4–1. DSM-5 Criteria for Cannabis Use Disorder

A. A problematic pattern of cannabis use leading to clinically significant impairment or distress, as manifested by at least two of the following, occurring within a 12-month period:

1. Cannabis is often taken in larger amounts or over a longer period than was intended.
2. There is a persistent desire or unsuccessful efforts to cut down or control cannabis use.
3. A great deal of time is spent in activities necessary to obtain cannabis, use cannabis, or recover from its effects.
4. Craving, or a strong desire or urge to use cannabis.
5. Recurrent cannabis use resulting in a failure to fulfill major role obligations at work, school, or home.
6. Continued cannabis use despite having persistent or recurrent social or interpersonal problems caused or exacerbated by the effects of cannabis.
7. Important social, occupational, or recreational activities are given up or reduced because of cannabis use.
8. Recurrent cannabis use in situations in which it is physically hazardous.
9. Cannabis use is continued despite knowledge of having a persistent or recurrent physical or psychological problem that is likely to have been caused or exacerbated by cannabis.

10. Tolerance, as defined by either of the following:
    a. A need for markedly increased amounts of cannabis to achieve intoxication or desired effect.
    b. Markedly diminished effect with continued use of the same amount of cannabis.
11. Withdrawal, as manifested by either of the following:
    a. The characteristic withdrawal syndrome for cannabis (refer to Criteria A and B of the criteria set for cannabis withdrawal, DSM-5 pp. 517–518).
    b. Cannabis (or a closely related substance) is taken to relieve or avoid withdrawal symptoms.

Specify if:

In early remission: After full criteria for cannabis use disorder were previously met, none of the criteria for cannabis use disorder have been met for at least 3 months but for less than 12 months (with the exception that Criterion A4, "Craving, or a strong desire or urge to use cannabis," may be met).

In sustained remission: After full criteria for cannabis use disorder were previously met, none of the criteria for cannabis use disorder have been met at any time during a period of 12 months or longer (with the exception that Criterion A4, "Craving, or a strong desire or urge to use cannabis," may be present).

Specify if:

In a controlled environment: This additional specifier is used if the individual is in an environment where access to cannabis is restricted.

Code based on current severity: Note for ICD-10-CM codes: If a cannabis intoxication, cannabis withdrawal, or another cannabis-induced mental disorder is also present, do not use the codes below for cannabis use disorder. Instead, the comorbid cannabis use disorder is indicated in the 4th character of the cannabis-induced disorder code (see the coding note for cannabis intoxication, cannabis withdrawal, or a specific cannabis-induced mental disorder). For example, if there is comorbid cannabis-induced anxiety disorder and cannabis use disorder, only the cannabis-induced anxiety disorder code is given, with the 4th character indicating whether the comorbid cannabis use disorder is mild, moderate, or severe: F12.180 for mild cannabis use disorder with cannabis-induced anxiety disorder or F12.280 for a moderate or severe cannabis use disorder with cannabis-induced anxiety disorder.

Specify current severity:

305.20 (F12.10) Mild: Presence of 2–3 symptoms.
304.30 (F12.20) Moderate: Presence of 4–5 symptoms.
304.30 (F12.20) Severe: Presence of 6 or more symptoms.

Source. Reprinted from the *Diagnostic and Statistical Manual of Mental Disorders,* 5th Edition, Washington, DC, American Psychiatric Association, 2013. Used with permission. Copyright © 2013 American Psychiatric Association.

Popular Terminology of Cannabis

Cannabis has achieved widespread popularity among many cultural groups. There are innumerable examples of cannabis use in mainstream print and television media. Some of the more common street names for cannabis use are pot, weed, mary jane, reefer, ganja, dube, grass, herb, chronic, and roach.

Psychopharmacology of Cannabis

Most cannabis is smoked and absorbed through the lungs and distributed throughout the body in fatty tissue for slow release. The psychoactive ingredient of cannabis, Δ-9-tetrahydrocannabinol (THC), crosses the blood-brain barrier and binds to endogenous G-protein-coupled cannabinoid receptors known as CB1, which are present throughout the brain. It is thought that THC modulates the mesolimbic dopamine reward system, leading to the positive psychoactive effects of the drug. Desensitization and tolerance develop in typical neurochemical fashion and lead to an uncomfortable withdrawal syndrome when abstinence occurs in a heavy user. It is thought that the THC content in commercially available marijuana has increased in the past 50 years from 1%–5% to 10%–15%.

Cannabis Intoxication

The psychoactive effects of cannabis intoxication (see Box 4–2) occur within minutes if the drug is inhaled and within hours if cannabis is ingested, often in the form of baked goods. Predicting clinical effects on the basis of dosage is challenging because of the illegal nature of cannabis and the wide variance in patient tolerance and metabolism rates. Most patients feel clinical effects of intoxication for up to 4 hours after cannabis use. Commonly reported effects of cannabis intoxication include feeling "high" with mild euphoria, anxiolysis, and elevated mood.

Not surprisingly, some cannabis users (often first-time users) report unpleasant feelings such as anxiety, panic, paranoia, psychosis, and dysphoria. Physical effects of cannabis intoxication include hypertension, tachypnea, increased appetite, conjunctival injection, and xerostomia (dry mouth).

Management of Cannabis Intoxication

Some patients may present to the emergency department with acute agitation that may have been precipitated by using cannabis, which is frequently "laced" or enhanced with a secondary psychoactive drug such as phencyclidine or cocaine. These patients may experience more severe symptoms such as psychosis, psychomotor agitation, paranoia, severe dysphoria, and heart palpitations. Treatment includes typical strategies such as limiting environmental stimuli in a quiet, dark room and psychopharmacological sedation with benzodiazepines (such as lorazepam) and antipsychotics (such as haloperidol or risperidone).

Box 4–2. DSM-5 Criteria for Cannabis Intoxication

A. Recent use of cannabis.
B. Clinically significant problematic behavioral or psychological changes (e.g., impaired motor coordination, euphoria, anxiety, sensation of slowed time, impaired judgment, social withdrawal) that developed during, or shortly after, cannabis use.
C. Two (or more) of the following signs or symptoms developing within 2 hours of cannabis use:
   1. Conjunctival injection.
   2. Increased appetite.
   3. Dry mouth.
   4. Tachycardia.
D. The signs or symptoms are not attributable to another medical condition and are not better explained by another mental disorder, including intoxication with another substance.

Specify if:

With perceptual disturbances: Hallucinations with intact reality testing or auditory, visual, or tactile illusions occur in the absence of a delirium.

Coding note: The ICD-9-CM code is **292.89.** The ICD-10-CM code depends on whether or not there is a comorbid cannabis use disorder and whether or not there are perceptual disturbances.

For cannabis intoxication, without perceptual disturbances: If a mild cannabis use disorder is comorbid, the ICD-10-CM code is **F12.129,** and if a moderate or severe cannabis use disorder is comorbid, the ICD-10-CM code is **F12.229.** If there is no comorbid cannabis use disorder, then the ICD-10-CM code is **F12.929.**

For cannabis intoxication, with perceptual disturbances: If a mild cannabis use disorder is comorbid, the ICD-10-CM code is **F12.122,** and if a moderate or severe cannabis use disorder is comorbid, the ICD-10-CM code is **F12.222.** If there is no comorbid cannabis use disorder, then the ICD-10-CM code is **F12.922.**

Source. Reprinted from the *Diagnostic and Statistical Manual of Mental Disorders,* 5th Edition, Washington, DC, American Psychiatric Association, 2013. Used with permission. Copyright © 2013 American Psychiatric Association.

Demographic Predictors of Cannabis Use Disorder

Many adolescents and young adults experiment with cannabis during their youth. The overwhelming majority of them do not develop cannabis use disorders. Longitudinal studies have revealed that 1%–2% of adolescents and young adults eventually develop cannabis use disorders (von Sydow et al. 2001).

An Australian study revealed risk factors for continued cannabis use as male sex, frequent use, early age of onset, using cannabis to reduce negative feelings, and other illegal drug use (Swift et al. 2000). The highest-risk age for developing cannabis use disorders is age 18.

The "Gateway Drug" Theory

Many researchers have theorized that although cannabis may not be profoundly dangerous in and of itself, it may lead to sequential use of more dangerous substances such as cocaine and opioids (Kaminer 2008). The old adage of "nobody ever starts out as a crack addict" comes to mind. To date, cannabis has not been definitely proven to be a "gateway drug," although this type of research is notoriously difficult to perform given concurrent substance use and co-occurring psychiatric disorders.

Medical Effects of Cannabis Use

Much has been written about the possible unhealthy medical effects of cannabis use. Some studies have shown very little medical impact, typically among low to moderate cannabis users. There is no consensus among epidemiologists and cancer researchers regarding the effect of cannabis use on cancer (Hashibe et al. 2005). Regarding the long-term neurocognitive defects of cannabis use, a 2003 meta-analysis and 1999 epidemiological study found no evidence that cannabis causes long-term effects (Grant et al. 2003). However, a large prospective 2012 study testing the association between persistent cannabis use and long-term neuropsychological decline showed a significant decrease in IQ points even after controlling for education levels (Meier et al. 2012). The decrease was particularly prominent in patients who developed cannabis use disorders as adolescents. As countries debate the potential legalization of cannabis, continued studies regarding long-term neurocognitive effects will be an important component of the discussion.

Psychiatric Effects of Cannabis Use

Many studies have demonstrated the negative effect of cannabis use on psychiatric health. A 2007 systematic review published in *The Lancet* demonstrated that there was a significantly increased risk of psychosis among cannabis users compared with noncannabis users (Moore et al. 2007). Among patients diagnosed with schizophrenia, the onset of psychosis occurred earlier among those who used cannabis. Cannabis has not been shown to induce depression.

Short-Term Neurocognitive Effects of Cannabis Use

No reported deaths have been directly attributed to intoxication with cannabis itself, although intoxication with cannabis has resulted in motor vehicle fatalities due to impaired attention and concentration as well as accidental drug overdoses from other drugs, resulting in death. Among drivers, those using cannabis are up to seven times more likely to be responsible for accidents compared with nonusing drivers (Leggett and United Nations Office on Drugs and Crime 2006). The duration of psychomotor delay associated with cannabis intoxication far exceeds the pleasurable "high" associated with cannabis, sometimes to as much as 24 hours after ingestion. One study among pilots showed impaired flight simulation performance 24 hours after smoking cannabis. Of more concern is the fact that only one of the pilots in the study was aware that he was still impaired; the remaining eight pilots felt that they were fine (Leirer et al. 1991).

Amotivational Syndrome

Much has been written about whether cannabis use is associated with a condition known as *amotivational syndrome.* At present, it is not clearly established whether cannabis use itself can specifically induce an amotivational syndrome. Although many individuals with an amotivational syndrome have a concurrent cannabis use disorder, controlling research studies for other risk factors such as co-occurring depression and demographic-related aspirations remains much more difficult.

Cannabis use among children and young adults has been associated with dropping out of school, use of other illegal drugs, increased criminal behavior, and unemployment. There have been studies of twins who are discordant for cannabis use that have indicated that when the twin using cannabis is able to achieve abstinence, sociodemographic indicators seem to return to the level of the non-cannabis-abusing twin (Elkashef et al. 2008).

Cannabis Withdrawal Syndrome

Much has also been written about the existence, or not, of a cannabis withdrawal syndrome. The newly released DSM-5 (American Psychiatric Association 2013) includes a definition for cannabis withdrawal syndrome (Box 4–3). The World Health Organization's (1992) International Classification of Diseases, 10th Revision (ICD-10) also endorses the existence of a cannabis withdrawal syndrome. Like cocaine, stimulant, and opioid withdrawal, cannabis withdrawal syndrome, although uncomfortable, is not life threatening.

Signs of cannabis withdrawal (within 2 days of abstinence) include fatigue, hypersomnolence, irritability, psychomotor retardation, decreased appetite or weight loss, depression and anxiety, and physical symptoms such as tremors, diaphoresis, fever, headache, and chills. Withdrawal symptoms tend to resolve after 3 weeks of abstinence.

Treatment of Cannabis Use Disorders

Treatment options for cannabis use disorders range from residential treatment to brief outpatient counseling. There is no clinically dangerous withdrawal syndrome from cannabis, so there is no role for detoxification. Often, patients with a cannabis use disorder have a concurrent dependence on another substance that may be the primary reason for them to seek treatment; it is important to recognize that cannabis disorders should be treated at the same time as the other substances. Harm reduction–based treatment modalities typically employed at methadone-based opiate agonist programs sometimes direct little effort toward cannabis disorders given their widespread prevalence. This approach remains controversial in the addiction medicine community. Abstinence is the de facto end goal of nationally recognized cannabis treatment strategies. As patients approach eventual abstinence, it can be beneficial to employ harm reduction techniques if abstinence is not achievable in the short term. Patients may set goals such as avoiding cannabis when they drive or operate heavy machinery. They can also agree to use cannabis only during the weekends or evenings.

Box 4–3. DSM-5 Criteria for Cannabis Withdrawal **292.0 (F12.288)**

A. Cessation of cannabis use that has been heavy and prolonged (i.e., usually daily or almost daily use over a period of at least a few months).
B. Three (or more) of the following signs and symptoms develop within approximately 1 week after Criterion A:
   1. Irritability, anger, or aggression.
   2. Nervousness or anxiety.
   3. Sleep difficulty (e.g., insomnia, disturbing dreams).
   4. Decreased appetite or weight loss.
   5. Restlessness.
   6. Depressed mood.
   7. At least one of the following physical symptoms causing significant discomfort: abdominal pain, shakiness/tremors, sweating, fever, chills, or headache.
C. The signs or symptoms in Criterion B cause clinically significant distress or impairment in social, occupational, or other important areas of functioning.
D. The signs or symptoms are not attributable to another medical condition and are not better explained by another mental disorder, including intoxication or withdrawal from another substance.

Coding note: The ICD-9-CM code is 292.0. The ICD-10-CM code for cannabis withdrawal is F12.288. Note that the ICD-10-CM code indicates the comorbid presence of a moderate or severe cannabis use disorder, reflecting the fact that cannabis withdrawal can only occur in the presence of a moderate or severe cannabis use disorder. It is not permissible to code a comorbid mild cannabis use disorder with cannabis withdrawal.

Source. Reprinted from the *Diagnostic and Statistical Manual of Mental Disorders,* 5th Edition, Washington, DC, American Psychiatric Association, 2013. Used with permission. Copyright © 2013 American Psychiatric Association.

Psychosocial Education

The gold standard for treating cannabis use disorders remains psychosocial interventions such as psychotherapy, motivational interviewing, and group therapy. Studies have suggested that psychotherapy is more likely to result in reduced cannabis use rather than full abstinence. Motivational interviewing, cognitive-behavior therapy, family therapy, and group therapy have all been shown to be efficacious in reducing cannabis use, although one particular approach has not been found to be better than others. Some programs have researched voucher incentives (typically monetary rewards) for continued abstinence and have shown increased success compared with nonvoucher programs. This type of approach, while notable, has obvious shortcomings when applied to society at large because of limited resources.

Pharmacotherapy for Cannabis Use Disorders

Antidepressants

There have been several randomized controlled trials examining the role of nefazodone or bupropion. They failed to show any efficacy regarding cannabis use, cannabis dependence severity, or cannabis withdrawal symptoms (Elkashef et al. 2008).

Acetylcysteine

Limited data from one trial suggest that *N*-acetylcysteine can be helpful in improving abstinence rates in the adolescent population. It is thought that *N*-acetylcysteine may modulate glutamate production in the nucleus accumbens. Future studies must be performed before this can be routinely recommended in cannabis use disorders (Gray et al. 2012).

Mood Stabilizers

Studies with divalproex have failed to show efficacy for cannabis use disorders (Haney et al. 2004).

Cannabis Agonist Therapy

Several commercially available cannabinoid agonist medications are approved by the U.S. Food and Drug Administration for pain and appetite stimulation in patients with AIDS as well as for chemotherapy-induced nausea for patients with cancer. These agents, specifically oral THC, have shown some success at decreasing withdrawal symptoms and cannabis craving during cannabis abstinence attempts. Other studies have shown benefit in preventing withdrawal symptoms and decreasing relapse by combining THC with lofexidine (a drug that is not available in the United States) (Haney et al. 2008). At present, cannabis agonist therapy is not approved for cannabis use disorders, although research is ongoing. Given the profound mortality and criminality differences between opioid abuse and cannabis abuse, it is unlikely that agonist therapy for cannabis abuse would gain significant health policy traction among legislators.

Natural Progression of Cannabis Use Disorders

Many people who meet criteria for cannabis use disorders during their college-age years are able to stop abusing cannabis successfully without professional intervention. This reality can sometimes undermine cannabis use disorder treatment because the disorder may seem illegitimate or "easy to beat" and not worthy of professional help. Unfortunately, once patients have abused cannabis for many years, their likelihood for long-term abstinence is significantly decreased. Among patients who had used cannabis regularly for up to 15 years, 50% returned to regular use after a 14-week outpatient treatment program (Swift et al. 2000). Lack of perceived physical risk with cannabis appears to be a significant obstacle to abstinence efforts among cannabis abusers.

Drug Monitoring for Cannabis During Treatment

As with any substance use disorder, it is important to monitor the patient's response to therapy. "Trust but verify" is the oft-repeated mantra in many addiction medicine clinics. Because the signs and symptoms of cannabis use disorders can often mimic other substance use disorders and psychiatric diseases, objective drug testing is an indispensable component of evaluation and treatment. Blood, urine, oral swabs, and hair can all be tested for cannabis compounds. Although some forensic and government organizations use advanced collecting techniques, urine testing remains the most widely available and inexpensive method for screening of cannabis use. The lipophilic properties of cannabis generate slow release into body fluids such that urine can yield a positive rest result for cannabis several months after cessation of use for a heavy user and up to 10 days after use for a casual user. Despite what many patients may protest about the existence of false-positive tests, there is no possibility of this when modern testing techniques are employed.

Prevention of Cannabis Use Disorders

There has been significant research done on how best to prevent future cannabis use among school-age children. One meta-analysis of four prior studies found that among 6th- and 7th-grade students, an active intervention significantly reduced follow-up assessments of cannabis use at 1, 2, 5, and 6 years after the intervention (Elkashef et al. 2008). It remains unclear what role cannabis legalization campaigns will have on future cannabis use disorders among young people.

Clinical Case 1

Derrick is a 23-year-old black male with a 5-year history of cannabis dependence. He reported smoking 5–10 marijuana blunts a day for the past 3 years. He reported that his first use was at age 18 at a party during his freshman year at a prestigious private university in the Northeast. Derrick said he liked the social aspect of smoking blunts, and it relieved the social anxiety he had had for most of his life. In addition, Derrick thought smoking pot enhanced the sound of music, allowing him to empathize better with the messages rappers conveyed in their songs. Even though there were no immediate consequences for smoking, Derrick began rationalizing his use of marijuana because he did not smoke every day: "I only smoke trees[1] with my friends on weekends, and it's not interfering with my class work." However, over time, Derrick's tolerance and frequency gradually increased from just on the weekend to a couple of days during the week to daily use.

Derrick's frequency of use increased as his class attendance and grades decreased. He was placed on academic probation but still was unable to make it to class because of low motivation and energy; he was asked to leave the school for poor academic performance. On returning home, Derrick began selling pot to support his addiction and supplement his income. Derrick spent most of his days sleeping late, smoking, selling pot, and going to various nightclubs. Notably, his illegal activities increased and he began to deal prescription drugs. He became well known among New York City's nightlife crowd. Subsequently, he was arrested and charged with possession of a controlled substance with intent to sell and deliver. Derrick received an indeterminate sentence of 4–8 years in a New York State prison and is not eligible for parole until 2017.

Although Derrick's story is tragic, while in prison he will be evaluated psychologically and possibly referred to treatment for substance abuse and mental health services. Contrary to the popular belief that marijuana is harmless, it can be as devastating as any other substance. According to Derrick, "if I'd known what smoking weed would do to me, I would have thought twice when that blunt was passed to me 5 years ago. For the next 4 and a half years I am reminded of the choice I made, rather, the lack of choice."

Clinical Case 2

In the 9th grade, Dave was a high-achieving student with a variety of extracurricular pursuits. He had been popular with his friends; excelled at tennis, baseball, and soccer; and enjoyed reading, movies, and travel with his parents. By all accounts, he was a good kid, and his parents remembered expecting big things from him as he progressed through high school. Dave remembered his first high-school party at a posh apartment in Manhattan; the host's parents had gone out of town for the weekend, and it seemed as though the entire school had congregated in the house. Alcohol, tobacco, and marijuana were passed around, and Dave, like almost everyone there, tried each product.

A few months later Dave had begun smoking marijuana almost every weekend. As he recalled, "it didn't really change anything; it's just what we all did." Dave had achieved decent grades and was accepted to an elite university on the East Coast. Once college began, however, things started to go downhill. He re-

[1]A slang term used to describe marijuana that originated in Brooklyn, New York, in 1994.

membered drinking "like any typical college kid," usually in binge episodes at fraternity parties. He did not enjoy hangovers, so he rarely drank during the week because he had to get up and attend classes. However, by his junior year he was smoking marijuana almost every night before bed and many days before class. He was quick to mention that his grades did not seem to be affected. His health was normal, he had friends, and everything seemed okay.

As college graduation approached, many of Dave's friends were busy making plans for graduate school or employment. Because of the prestige of Dave's school, many of his classmates were interviewing at well-known banks and consulting firms in Manhattan. As he recalled, "I guess I just remember not even filling out the applications; I think I just wanted to chill." He graduated and moved back to New York City and back into his old bedroom in his parents' apartment building. He found work as a waiter at a trendy restaurant on the Lower East Side of Manhattan. Because of what he perceived as a monotonous job, he smoked marijuana before every shift. Now 22 years old, Dave was smoking marijuana every day in the morning, afternoon, and evening. Accessing marijuana was never a problem for Dave, and he was never arrested for possession. As he put it later, "nobody cares if you smoke weed in the city; it just isn't a big deal."

I first met Dave when he was 30 and had entered an inpatient drug and alcohol rehabilitation center in New York City for cannabis abuse and dependence. Dave mentioned that he had tried other illegal substances such as cocaine (once) and hallucinogenic mushrooms (several times). He had never tried illegal opioids or methamphetamines. He drinks socially (2–3 beers per week with friends) and smokes one pack of tobacco cigarettes per day. Dave holds a combined undergraduate degree in comparative literature and economics from one of America's most prestigious universities, yet he has never held a job other than as a waiter and has been unemployed for the past 3 years. As he put it, "all of my buddies from college stopped smoking weed; I just couldn't quit."

Dave completed a 30-day inpatient residential treatment program specializing in both group and individual psychotherapy rooted in motivational interviewing techniques. His treatment course was unremarkable, and he was discharged home on no medications. At 90 days after discharge he was endorsing full abstinence, and several negative urine toxicology tests corroborated his reports. He has found full-time employment at a bookstore and is enrolling in graduate classes to become a high school teacher. He no longer smokes cigarettes and is training for the New York City Marathon.

Discussion

Dave and Derrick's stories are likely to resonate for several reasons with many patients and clinical providers. Their introduction to cannabis occurred in typical fashion, at a high school party. The growth of their addiction was insidious and barely noticeable until they were many years into it. They experienced no physical sequelae from cannabis use and remained fairly healthy into early adulthood. Aside from some exercise intolerance likely related to years of cigarette smoking, Dave was a healthy young man. He was never involved with the criminal justice system and had never been diagnosed with a mental health disorder other than cannabis abuse and dependence. Despite all that, Dave and Derrick would be the first to admit that cannabis ruined a large portion of their lives. Dave spent the entirety of his young adulthood under the influence of cannabis. Derrick remains incarcerated. Since age 22 Dave was "high" for every wedding he attended, every relationship he was ever in, and every meal he had ever eaten. As he says, "there was no such thing as non-high Dave."

Experimentation with marijuana usually occurs during early to late adolescence, a developmental stage that is filled with social pressures of fitting in and how one is viewed. Derrick stated that smoking pot helped to relieve the social anxiety he had had for most of his life. Even though he has no family history of mental illness or mental health treatment, Derrick may have undiagnosed generalized anxiety disorder. Last, daily pot use decreases an individual's motivation, ambitions, or drive toward achieving personal goals. Consequently, pot use can progress to illicit drug use (e.g., heroin, oxycodone, crack, and alprazolam) and maladaptive behaviors to maintain and support one's addiction.

Pot is a gateway drug in multiple ways; for instance, shy and insecure youths smoking with others can initiate contact with their peers. It allows them to establish their own identity—one that may conflict with the one assigned by their family of origin. More importantly, smoking pot can be used to self-medicate an undiagnosed mental health disorder.

Recognizing cannabis use disorders among patients, particularly young adults, is notoriously difficult. It is challenging to tease out "normal young adult behavior" from potential addiction. As stated earlier, the likelihood is that most cannabis users will spontaneously recover. Many researchers have postulated that "real life" events such as marriage, career advancement, and parenthood tend to have the positive effect of curing cannabis abuse. Unfortunately, there will always be people like Dave and Derrick, and they deserve our continued professional care.

Key Points

- The psychoactive ingredient of cannabis is Δ-9-tetrahydrocannabinol (THC). THC binds to endogenous G-protein coupled cannabinoid receptors known as CB1 that are present throughout the brain.
- Treatment for cannabis intoxication includes limiting environmental stimuli in a quiet, dark room as well as psychopharmacological sedation with benzodiazepines and antipsychotics.
- Patients who continually use cannabis are more likely to abuse other psychoactive substances than those who do not use cannabis.

- Although many studies have demonstrated the negative effect of cannabis use on psychiatric health, no long-term neurocognitive defects have been proven.
- Cannabis use disorder may lead to sequential use of more dangerous substances such as cocaine and opiates.
- Cannabis use among children and young adults has been associated with dropping out of school, use of other illegal drugs, increased criminal behavior, and unemployment.
- No reported deaths have been directly attributed to intoxication with cannabis. However, intoxication with cannabis has resulted in motor vehicle fatalities due to impaired concentration.
- Treatment options for cannabis use disorders range from residential treatment to brief outpatient counseling.
- Once patients have abused cannabis for many years, their likelihood for long-term abstinence is significantly decreased.

References

American Psychiatric Association: Diagnostic and Statistical Manual of Mental Disorders, 5th Edition. Washington, DC, American Psychiatric Association, 2013

Conway KP, Compton W, Stinson FS, et al: Lifetime comorbidity of DSM-IV mood and anxiety disorders and specific drug use disorders: results from the National Epidemiologic Survey on Alcohol and Related Conditions. J Clin Psychiatry 67:247–257, 2006

Dutra L, Stathopoulou G, Basden SL, et al: A meta-analytic review of psychosocial interventions for substance use disorders. Am J Psychiatry 165:179–187, 2008

Elkashef A, Vocci F, Huestis M, et al: Marijuana neurobiology and treatment. Subst Abus 29:17–29, 2008

Grant I, Gonzalez R, Carey CL, et al: Non-acute (residual) neurocognitive effects of cannabis use: a meta-analytic study. J Int Neuropsychol Soc 9:679–689, 2003

Gray KM, Carpenter MJ, Baker NL, et al: A double-blind randomized controlled trial of *N*-acetylcysteine in cannabis-dependent adolescents. Am J Psychiatry 169:805–812, 2012

Haney M, Hart CL, Vosburg SK, et al: Marijuana withdrawal in humans: effects of oral THC or divalproex. Neuropsychopharmacology 29:158–170, 2004

Haney M, Hart CL, Vosburg SK, et al: Effects of THC and lofexidine in a human laboratory model of marijuana withdrawal and relapse. Psychopharmacology (Berl) 197:157–168, 2008

Hashibe M, Straif K, Tashkin DP, et al: Epidemiologic review of marijuana use and cancer risk. Alcohol 35:265–275, 2005

Kaminer Y: Adolescent substance abuse, in The American Psychiatric Publishing Textbook of Substance Abuse Treatment, 4th Edition. Edited by Galanter M, Kleber HD. Washington, DC, American Psychiatric Publishing, 2008, pp 527–545

Leggett T, United Nations Office on Drugs and Crime: A review of the world cannabis situation. Bull Narc 58:1–155, 2006

Leirer VO, Yesavage JA, Morrow DG: Marijuana carry-over effects on aircraft pilot performance. Aviat Space Environ Med 62:221–227, 1991

Meier M, Caspi A, Ambler A, et al: Persistent cannabis users show neuropsychological decline from childhood to midlife. Proc Natl Acad Sci 109:E2657–E2664, 2012

Moore TH, Zammit S, Lingford-Hughes A, et al: Cannabis use and risk of psychotic or affective mental health outcomes: a systematic review. Lancet 370:319–328, 2007

Swift W, Hall W, Copeland J: One year follow-up of cannabis dependence among long-term users in Sydney, Australia. Drug Alcohol Depend 59:309–318, 2000

von Sydow K, Lieb R, Pfister H, et al: The natural course of cannabis use, abuse and dependence over four years: a longitudinal community study of adolescents and young adults. Drug Alcohol Depend 64:347–361, 2001

World Health Organization: International Statistical Classification of Diseases and Related Health Problems, 10th Revision. Geneva, Switzerland, World Health Organization, 1992

Questions

4.1 Jenny presents to you as her primary care physician and reveals a nearly 3-year-long dependence on cannabis. She is concerned because she and her husband Craig are planning to start a family, and she asks your advice about which treatment strategy you might recommend. Which of the following is the most appropriate treatment for Jenny?

A. Start bupropion at 150 mg/day for 2 weeks and then increase to 300 mg/day for an 8-week course.
B. Explain to Jenny that cannabis use has not been associated with any medical problems and provide reassurance.
C. Refer Jenny to a local substance abuse facility for an intake appointment for psychosocial counseling.
D. Send Jenny to a local psychiatrist for further evaluation.

The correct answer is C.

A is incorrect because antidepressants such as bupropion have not been shown to be beneficial for cannabis abuse. B is incorrect because although cannabis abuse has not been associated with any medical problems, it causes a wide arrange of social problems. D is incorrect because patients often reveal substance abuse problems after many months or years of agonizing self-deception. Many patients are profoundly ambivalent regarding their disease, and the clinician must quickly recognize a motivated patient. Sending her to a psychiatrist will delay her entry into treatment and may lead her to lose motivation.

4.2 Doug is a 35-year-old successful computer programmer who has recently accepted a contract position with NASA. Part of his pre-employment screening involves a urine drug screen in 1 month, and he is concerned that he will fail it because he has abused cannabis for many years. He asks you about what you might recommend for "detoxing" from cannabis. Which of the following is the best advice for Doug?

A. Explain to Doug that he should stop smoking cannabis immediately and purchase an over-the-counter multivitamin to help "cleanse" the cannabis from his body. You anticipate he will pass the test.
B. Explain to Doug that he has cannabis withdrawal syndrome. Advise that he stop cannabis and recommend supportive care for any symptoms that may develop. Do not provide any guidance on the test.
C. Tell Doug to smoke decreasing amounts of cannabis each day so that he can "come down slowly" from the drug with the expectation that he can be fully abstinent for 1 week prior to his test.
D. Prescribe *N*-acetylcysteine to Doug at 1,200 mg twice daily for a 4-week course. Recommend that he stay "extra hydrated" before the urine test.

The correct answer is B.

A is incorrect because multivitamins and other commercially available "detox" supplements have not been approved by the U.S. Food and Drug Administration for any condition. As a chronic, heavy user of cannabis for many years, Doug is actually at significant risk for failing his urine test because these types of users can remain positive for cannabis on urine tests for several months after abstinence. C is incorrect because cannabis withdrawal does not respond to decreased titration of a daily dose. D is incorrect because *N*-acetylcysteine is used only as an augmentative addition to ongoing psychosocial counseling. Furthermore, there is no role for hydration before a urine test.

4.3 Which of the following modalities have been proven to be *most* effective for the treatment of cannabis use disorders?

A. Motivational interviewing.
B. Group counseling.
C. Psychosocial education.
D. Selective serotonin reuptake inhibitors.
E. Options A, B, and C are all equivalent in their success.

The correct answer is E.

D is incorrect because there is no role for antidepressants in the treatment of cannabis use disorders.

CHAPTER 5

Hallucinogens

The Mind Field of Oswald: A Case of Hallucinogen Intoxication

Elias Dakwar, M.D.

THE term *hallucinogen* designates a diverse group of substances whose primary effects are unique alterations in perception, experience, and consciousness. Before we review the neurobiology and phenomenology of these effects, it is worth emphasizing that hallucinogens, despite their name, rarely engender hallucinations (or sensory phenomena that are experienced as real although lacking a referent in reality). This has led to other names being proposed for this drug class, such as psychedelic (mind manifesting), phantasticant (fantasy inducing), oneirogen (dream generating), and deliriant. *Hallucinogen* (from the Latin *alucinor:* mental wandering or dreaming) remains the most widely used term for these substances in medical settings, and we will employ it here, its limitations notwithstanding.

The background to this chapter's clinical case will be lengthier than that of other chapters to ensure that the complexities and nuances of this unique drug class are appreciated. This will allow us to better understand the subtle clinical challenges that exist in the case of Oswald, which is modeled on an encounter with an actual patient. The background will also include a brief cultural history of hallucinogen use among preindustrial groups and in the United States of the

1960s because this will be helpful for understanding the sociocultural salience of hallucinogens. As we will see later with Oswald, sociocultural factors constitute an important aspect of hallucinogen use and can provide valuable guidance on how to clinically approach it.

Classifications and Effects

Hallucinogens are classified by 1) their molecular structure or 2) their direct neurobiological activity (Bakalar and Grinspoon 1997). The two most common structural subgroups are indoles and phenethylamines. Indoles include lysergic acid diethylamide (LSD), dimethyltryptamine (DMT), psilocybin, ibogaine, and harmaline. Phenethylamines include naturally occurring compounds such as mescaline as well as an ever-expanding number of synthetic variations, such as 4-bromo-2,5-dimethoxyphenethylamine (2C-B), 3,4-methylenedioxy-*N*-methylamphetamine (MDMA), 3,4-methylenedioxyamphetamine (MDA), and 2,5-dimethoxy-4-methylamphetamine (DOM).

Classical hallucinogens work by direct agonism of the 5-HT_{2A} serotonin receptor and include psilocybin, LSD, mescaline, and DMT. Although these compounds share neurobiological activity, they come from quite diverse sources: psilocybin can be isolated from a mushroom; DMT is found in a South American vine and is also endogenously elaborated by the pineal gland; mescaline derives from a cactus in the American Southwest; and LSD is an ergot derivative that can be synthesized in a laboratory.

Hallucinogens may also exert their psychoactive effects by serotonin release or nonspecific serotonin receptor activation, as in the case of MDMA ("ecstasy" or "Molly"‘) and some phenethylamines; by *N*-methyl-D-aspartate (NMDA) receptor or glutamatergic modulation, such as ketamine, phencyclidine, and other dissociative anesthetics; by cannabinoid receptor activation; and by κ receptor agonism, as occurs with *Salvia divinorum*. These mechanisms are by no means exhaustive; there are other compounds (e.g., nitrous oxide and the fly agaric mushroom) that work by quite different mechanisms. Interestingly, recent research suggests that hallucinogens, despite their apparent differences in neurobiological activity, work by a common final pathway of prefrontal glutamatergic modulation (Vollenweider and Kometer 2010).

The psychoactive effects of these different compounds can be markedly different (see Boxes 5–1 and 5–2). Even compounds from the same subgroup (e.g., DMT and psilocybin) can be quite dissimilar. It is therefore beyond the purview of this chapter to provide a meticulous examination of the unique effects of each hallucinogen. Instead, we aim to describe all *potential* hallucinogenic effects. Classical hallucinogens are the subgroup that typically exhibits the widest range of these effects.

Box 5–1. DSM-5 Criteria for Phencyclidine Intoxication

A. Recent use of phencyclidine (or a pharmacologically similar substance).
B. Clinically significant problematic behavioral changes (e.g., belligerence, assaultiveness, impulsiveness, unpredictability, psychomotor agitation, impaired judgment) that developed during, or shortly after, phencyclidine use.
C. Within 1 hour, two (or more) of the following signs or symptoms:

Note: When the drug is smoked, "snorted," or used intravenously, the onset may be particularly rapid.

1. Vertical or horizontal nystagmus.
2. Hypertension or tachycardia.
3. Numbness or diminished responsiveness to pain.
4. Ataxia.
5. Dysarthria.
6. Muscle rigidity.
7. Seizures or coma.
8. Hyperacusis.

D. The signs or symptoms are not attributable to another medical condition and are not better explained by another mental disorder, including intoxication with another substance.

Coding note: The ICD-9-CM code is **292.89.** The ICD-10-CM code depends on whether there is a comorbid phencyclidine use disorder. If a mild phencyclidine use disorder is comorbid, the ICD-10-CM code is **F16.129,** and if a moderate or severe phencyclidine use disorder is comorbid, the ICD-10-CM code is **F16.229.** If there is no comorbid phencyclidine use disorder, then the ICD-10-CM code is **F16.929.**

Source. Reprinted from the *Diagnostic and Statistical Manual of Mental Disorders,* 5th Edition, Washington, DC, American Psychiatric Association, 2013. Used with permission. Copyright © 2013 American Psychiatric Association.

Hallucinogenic alterations can be grouped into three categories, all of which can be experienced concurrently. Most narratives offered by individuals who have undergone a hallucinogenic experience suggest a progression of effects in which one category of alterations is necessary for the next to emerge. The first and most basic are perceptual changes. These include an intensification of sensory phenomena; greater sensitivity to latent phenomena, such as patterns or textures ordinarily overlooked; changes in the perception of time or space; conflation of sensory modalities, as in synesthesia; the production of eidetic imagery, such as spirals, shapes, and arabesques; greater aesthetic appreciation; illusions; pseudo hallucinations (with intact reality testing); and an altered sense of the body.

Box 5–2. DSM-5 Criteria for Other Hallucinogen Intoxication

A. Recent use of a hallucinogen (other than phencyclidine).
B. Clinically significant problematic behavioral or psychological changes (e.g., marked anxiety or depression, ideas of reference, fear of "losing one's mind," paranoid ideation, impaired judgment) that developed during, or shortly after, hallucinogen use.
C. Perceptual changes occurring in a state of full wakefulness and alertness (e.g., subjective intensification of perceptions, depersonalization, derealization, illusions, hallucinations, synesthesias) that developed during, or shortly after, hallucinogen use.
D. Two (or more) of the following signs developing during, or shortly after, hallucinogen use:
   1. Pupillary dilation.
   2. Tachycardia.
   3. Sweating.
   4. Palpitations.
   5. Blurring of vision.
   6. Tremors.
   7. Incoordination.
E. The signs or symptoms are not attributable to another medical condition and are not better explained by another mental disorder, including intoxication with another substance.

Coding note: The ICD-9-CM code is **292.89.** The ICD-10-CM code depends on whether there is a comorbid hallucinogen use disorder. If a mild hallucinogen use disorder is comorbid, the ICD-10-CM code is **F16.129,** and if a moderate or severe hallucinogen use disorder is comorbid, the ICD-10-CM code is **F16.229.** If there is no comorbid hallucinogen use disorder, then the ICD-10-CM code is **F16.929.**

Source. Reprinted from the *Diagnostic and Statistical Manual of Mental Disorders,* 5th Edition, Washington, DC, American Psychiatric Association, 2013. Used with permission. Copyright © 2013 American Psychiatric Association.

The second category of alterations is experiential. These changes include alterations in mood (euphoria, hilarity, terror, or anxiety), altered relatedness to others (empathy, alienation, connectedness, or merging), philosophical or existential concerns, increased insight, dissociation, emergence of pseudo delusional or overvalued ideas (e.g., the world will end in the near future), suggestibility, resurgence of past or apparently resolved conflicts, and near-death or birth-like experiences.

Mystical or transpersonal experiences constitute the third category. These are experiences characterized by heightened spirituality or mysticism, similar in nature to those reported by mystics or religious figures throughout history. They can include a struggle or conflict of archetypal dimensions, a sense of life's fundamental absurdity, immersion in a total void, a sense of the sacred, spiritual ecstasy, spatiotemporal transcendence, nondiscursive understanding (e.g., knowledge beyond the pale of words or concepts), ego dissolution, an overwhelming sense of finiteness or sinfulness, identification with the divine, reincarnation, reevaluation of values, redemption, or metaphysical or cosmological speculation. Recent research with psilocybin suggests that the personal significance of such experiences can be enduring, with individuals continuing to report 1 year later that the experience was among the most important in their lives (Griffiths et al. 2006).

Anecdotal reports suggest that hallucinogenic alterations are shaped, to an extent, by the psychology, past experience, expectations or intentions, and attributes of the individual (the *set*), as well as by the environment (including other individuals or a guide if present) in which the experience occurs (the *setting*). The set and setting may also play a primary role with regard to whether the hallucinogen experience is pleasant and enriching ("a good trip") or dysphoric and upsetting ("a bad trip").

Cultural History

As is the case with many psychoactive substances, hallucinogens have been accorded an important, and sometimes sacramental, place in various cultural traditions (Bakalar and Grinspoon 1997). The unique profile of their effects, particularly in regard to producing mystical experience, has made them especially well suited to religious, initiation, or healing ceremonies. The fly agaric mushroom has an important role in Siberian shamanic rituals, and it has also been used in Scandinavia as a means to stimulate collective bloodlust and aggression just prior to entering battle. Certain African tribes continue to administer ibogaine for healing and spiritual divination to this day. Some scholarship, although possibly dubious, has further conjectured that the Eleusian mysteries in ancient Greece employed an ergot-derived hallucinogenic brew and that the heaven-sent drug Soma from the Vedic tradition was in fact a hallucinogenic mushroom.

Indigenous groups in the Americas have the most robust and diverse history in the world of incorporating hallucinogens into their rituals and ceremonies, likely because of the wealth of naturally occurring psychoactive substances in these continents. Tribes in Mexico, such as the Aztecs, have ritualized the use of psilocybin-containing mushrooms for thousands of years; peyote (mescaline) and salvia are also used by Mexican tribes; and DMT, in the form of ayahuasca or yage, is central to shamanic or religious ritual in various Amazonian groups. Although DMT and mescaline are illegal in the United States, they may be licitly used in their naturally occurring forms by members of certain tribes or religions that are recognized by the U.S. government as requiring these substances for proper worship.

This cultural background is important for understanding the reception of hallucinogens in the United States in the latter half of the twentieth century (Bakalar and Grinspoon 1997). Originally studied for their therapeutic capacity and, more covertly, as agents of chemical warfare, hallucinogens began to attract problematic public attention when they became associated with burgeoning youth movements, alternative lifestyles, and the counterculture in the late 1950s and 1960s. These negative associations were reinforced by the stigma that mescaline and psilocybin carried because of their identification with "primitive" indigenous groups and because of the apparent propensity of hallucinogens to provide immediate, personal, and enduring spiritual experience, which may have threatened the dominant Judeo-Christian system of institutionally mediated religious engagement. Even as studies were suggesting that LSD might be effective for treating alcoholism, hallucinogens were largely reclassified as illegal by the late 1960s, which brought medical research to a halt.

The criminalization of hallucinogens was buttressed by various claims for which there was no evidence but that nonetheless have managed to linger in the public consciousness (Sadock et al. 2009). These include concerns that hallucinogens cause chromosomal damage; that they create lasting psychotic disturbances in individuals without a preexisting vulnerability; that they lead to cognitive impairment with repeated use; that they lead to suicide, murder, or debauchery; or that they lead to schizotypal personality changes. Many of these claims contribute to the mystification that has surrounded these substances since the 1960s, which has sometimes precluded appropriate scientific and clinical understanding of them. However, this does not mean that hallucinogens are free of risk or that there is no reason for social concern.

Adverse Effects and Abuse

Recent U.S. polls indicate that hallucinogens are used most commonly in late adolescence and young adulthood, with up to 11% of 12th graders having used them at least once, and that their use is generally sporadic, clustered, or infrequent (Galanter and Kleber 2008). Even heavy users do not use more than two or three times per week. It is uncommon for hallucinogen use to persist beyond young adulthood. Barring atypical substances such as ketamine, nitrous oxide, certain phenethylamines, and cannabis (which was discussed in Chapter 4, "Cannabis"), hallucinogens do not create physiological dependence or tolerance, and dependence phenomena are rarely seen. Animal models of abuse liability suggest that classical hallucinogens do not present a risk for dependence; they are not self-administered, do not create conditioned place preference or physiological dependence, and do not lead to dopamine release from reward pathways (Bakalar and Grinspoon 1997; Galanter and Kleber 2008; Sadock et al. 2009).

What may be seen in humans, however, is hallucinogen abuse, where ill-considered use might lead to social, medical, or psychological impairment. Common adverse effects of hallucinogens include anxiety or dysphoria, circumscribed to the experience itself; loss of behavioral control, including passivity, disorganization, indecision, and suboptimal functioning, again during the period of acute effects; and more rarely, precipitation of enduring anxiety, affective, or psychotic disturbances in vulnerable individuals. A rare adverse phenomenon is the *flashback* (hallucinogen persisting perception disorder), which is characterized by sudden, impairing, and typically transient periods of perceptual alterations reminiscent of the hallucinogen experience but occurring well after acute effects have subsided (Box 5–3). The etiology of this phenomenon is not well understood; some psychopathologists conceptualize it as a posttraumatic reexperiencing of hallucinogen-related distress, whereas others conjecture that it represents a pathological manifestation of hallucinogen-induced neural plasticity. Hallucinogen abuse occurs when an individual continues to use hallucinogens despite repeatedly incurring any of the aforementioned adverse effects to the point of medical or psychosocial impairment.

The most serious hallucinogen-related adverse event occurs with MDMA. MDMA users may develop dangerously elevated body temperatures, which may in turn lead to cardiac and cerebral toxicity. The essential acute treatment is reducing the person's temperature.

Box 5–3. DSM-5 Criteria for Hallucinogen Persisting Perception Disorder **292.89 (F16.983)**

A. Following cessation of use of a hallucinogen, the reexperiencing of one or more of the perceptual symptoms that were experienced while intoxicated with the hallucinogen (e.g., geometric hallucinations, false perceptions of movement in the peripheral visual fields, flashes of color, intensified colors, trails of images of moving objects, positive afterimages, halos around objects, macropsia and micropsia).

B. The symptoms in Criterion A cause clinically significant distress or impairment in social, occupational, or other important areas of functioning.

C. The symptoms are not attributable to another medical condition (e.g., anatomical lesions and infections of the brain, visual epilepsies) and are not better explained by another mental disorder (e.g., delirium, major neurocognitive disorder, schizophrenia) or hypnopompic hallucinations.

Source. Reprinted from the *Diagnostic and Statistical Manual of Mental Disorders,* 5th Edition, Washington, DC, American Psychiatric Association, 2013. Used with permission. Copyright © 2013 American Psychiatric Association.

These adverse effects suggest the ways in which problematic hallucinogen use might come to clinical attention. Given the acute nature of most hallucinogen-related distress, a common setting for managing hallucinogen toxicity is the emergency department. Hallucinogen abuse, on the other hand, is most likely to present clinically in outpatient settings, when an individual (or concerned friends and family) finds that hallucinogen use is creating dysfunction in important domains. As mentioned earlier, certain hallucinogens (e.g., ketamine) may also lead to dependence. However, it is uncommon for individuals to seek treatment for problematic hallucinogen use or even to volunteer to health workers, unsolicited, their history of hallucinogen use—a not uncommon phenomenon with most cases of substance use. These clinical challenges, and how to go about addressing them, become clearer as we examine the following case.

Clinical Case

Oswald is a 22-year-old Caucasian man who was brought in no apparent distress to the emergency department of a large urban hospital by his parents, with whom he lived. He had no known history of medical or mental illness and no family history of psychiatric disorders and was taking no medications. His urine toxicology was negative for all drugs. Laboratory work, physical examination, and vital signs were unremarkable.

The patient's mother, an anxious woman in her early 40s, told the triage nurse that she was concerned that her son had taken a substance—she suspected some sort of psychedelic—that led him to start acting strangely. In particular, he had decided to adopt a completely plant based diet, had stopped shaving his face, was learning how to chant and play a hand drum, and had a newfound interest in what he termed "ecological interconnectedness" and "Gaia power." His mother reported that many of these changes were completely unprecedented and had begun about 2 weeks earlier when he returned home one morning "clearly having taken something powerful." She worried he may have used whatever it was at least one subsequent time. "He told me that there is no difference between God and himself a few days ago," she said. His father provided a similar history, noting that the patient had always been a good student "on track with a solid major [in business] to landing a nice job" but had decided halfway through senior year to take a year off after college to move back home and "find himself." The father, a sharply dressed bank manager, was concerned that his son, the elder of two boys, might be heading toward becoming "one of those directionless and irresponsible 20-somethings."

Oswald, however, thought that his parents were distorting recent events and "letting their egos ruin everything" by not allowing him to find "[his] own path." He was dressed in casual clothing and had been waiting impatiently on his gurney for the interview with his parents to conclude. He was well groomed, thin, and wore a short beard. He described his parents' account of a sudden shift in his personality and interests as incorrect. "I have always been interested in these things, even though I played the game so as to keep everyone off my back," he related. "I'm just not interested in playing the game anymore."

He acknowledged having experimented with various substances of abuse over the course of college, including cannabis, LSD, psilocybin, MDMA, and cocaine. His last use of cannabis occurred with friends 1 month prior, and his previous use had been one or two times a month over the past 3 years. He had used LSD twice 2 and 3 years prior at parties, psilocybin mushrooms once while hiking 1 year prior, MDMA several times during his junior year, and cocaine intranasally once at a party during his freshman year. He also drank several alcoholic drinks every weekend until 2 weeks prior, when he decided to stop "poisoning [his] body" and gave up alcohol completely. "All the other drugs I did because that's what you did, what everyone did. The acid and 'shrooms and E I liked, but I didn't choose to do them at the time, you know? I wasn't awake when I did them, I wasn't deliberate, not like I am now, not like with the shaman."

Two weeks prior, Oswald had decided to participate in an ayahuasca ceremony with an "urban shaman" he had been told about by friends. "When I heard about this, it was like something was calling to me. It was exactly what I had been looking for. I needed to wake up; I needed to see reality for what it was, without all the ego and layers getting in the way." The patient related that at his first meeting with the shaman, a white male social worker and artist in his mid-40s, he was been instructed to fast and prepare himself for a powerful spiritual experience. He did exactly as instructed, fasting after dinner for the afternoon ritual the following day and studying passages from the *Tao Te Ching* and the *Bhagavad Gita* that the shaman had designated for him. "I didn't understand everything I read, but those words totally planted a seed."

The ayahuasca ceremony occurred in a downtown apartment, and several other people, ranging in age from early 20s to late 50s, were also "initiates." After a group meditation, a preparatory talk, and some drumming and chanting led by the shaman, the group of initiates was given mugs of viscous black liquid to drink. Oswald asked if he could describe the experience in full detail, and after receiving an affirmative response, he said, "I wrote it down so I could remember every detail." He pulled a notebook out of his backpack and began to read:

I felt a little sick at first, as the shaman had said would happen, but I didn't throw up. And maybe an hour or so later, while laying down and waiting for the effects to kick in, I began to feel like I was floating. My skin was warm and wet. There was some kind of sticky dark liquid all around me. It seemed I was being swept along with a gentle stream. And the world was kind of hazy with underwater ripples. I could see shapes, flashes of images and faces. I could feel the history of the universe from the very beginning, but it was like history was compressed into solid state, the past and the future, everything that had ever existed and will ever exist mingled together. Was this the primordial mud? Time seemed to have stopped into a single moment, or perhaps it had expanded to include the past, present, and future simultaneously. My mind felt clear and alert, and I took it all in with eyes wide open, a rush of excitement going up and down my spine.

Pretty soon I heard a drumming sound, a heartbeat, boom boom boom, and my skin seemed to expand and contract with each beat. Everything felt like it was on the verge of bursting: the mud, the water, my electric brain. But maybe I was about to have a heart attack? I could actually feel my heart starting and stopping. I was scared that I was going to die, that I had finally gone too far and I was going to be punished somehow. I sensed that God was angry with me for some reason; maybe I was like that guy who flew too close to the sun. Or maybe I was greedy, always wanting more. I was terrified my heart would stop forever at any moment. Petrify. I could visualize it growing hard and black like a piece of coal. I remember thinking, I'm not sure why, "people want shiny diamonds so they turn their hearts into coal and die a thousand years."

But I took a deep breath and let it out for what seemed an eternity. Dying. Living again. I realized that breathing is living and dying: to exhale is to surrender yourself, and to inhale is to take in something new; every breath is death and rebirth. I was ecstatic with this discovery. So I let it all go, allowing the black liquid to fill my veins and brain, allowing the blood of the universe to be my blood. And I realized that the blood is eternal because it belongs to God. And I experienced it; I experienced God coursing through my vessels, giving me wisdom and love and understanding. This wasn't a God to be scared of but a God to celebrate.

Then the cycle of living and dying intensified. I went through a thousand forms, a thousand existences, and a thousand lifetimes. I became fascinated with the words *womb* and *tomb*, the secret links that exist between them, and the special way they fill the mouth with air coming from inside. I think I may have sung them out loud for a while. And I was transforming every second, living and dying in the blood of God. Each moment had a special lesson for me; things you read about in books like the *Bhagavad Gita* were actually happening to me. With the black river glistening all around me, I learned about compassion and pride and the thousand vanities of the ego. So many lessons and insights it would take a lifetime to write them all down. But everything came back to this: I learned that God is the only thing. I had never felt so fulfilled and happy.

I looked back at the life I had been living and I just wanted to laugh with tears in my eyes, laugh at how ignorant I had been, and cruel and stupid and sad too. I saw myself as some kind of robotic fool, and I remembered how, day in and day out, I would act out my preprogrammed routines. I had been stuck in myself for way too long while ignoring the living, pulsing world around me. But then I remembered a line from the readings I had been given, "The Tao that can be named is not the eternal Tao." And this line kept repeating in my head while my destiny flashed before my eyes. All the little signs when I was a kid and then growing up and then college: all these secret signs that I was heading in this direction. I was shivering with excitement and gratitude; the Tao had been with me all along. I was just too much in my head to see it. I was thinking too much, naming too much, instead of just being.

And here it was, God working in mysterious ways, bringing me back into reality using a path that I was bound to take, a shaman and ayahuasca and drums and all that. My path was full of these "mind fields," I realized, these things that are waiting for you so that they can surprise you, explode your reality and make room for what is really real. That was another phrase I think I had chanted: mind field. It seemed such a perfect expression. I me my mine mind field. I me mine....

I could have died then, and I would have been totally fine with it, because now I know there is no death, no birth, just a series of mind fields so that we can get closer to the divine river of Tao. But I was opening my eyes to life as if I was coming from another world, like a newborn baby. The ceremony was over, something like 10 hours had passed, and I felt brand new and old as the Earth itself at the same time. I was ready to get cracking; I didn't want to waste even a single second.

He finished reading and looked up excitedly. "See, the point is I finally had the courage and vision to do all those things I had wanted to do, everything I needed to do, without bothering about maintaining appearances or satisfying my parents. And that's why they're so pissed off: because I want to do things for myself."

He was then asked about further ayahuasca use, to which he responded,

> I didn't need the ayahuasca, by the way, and I don't plan on doing it again, even if I could afford another $700 session from my graduation money. The ayahuasca was like a door I needed to cross, but the point is getting to where I need to go, not the door itself. It could have been any other door, do you know what I mean? I'm done with ayahuasca, I don't need drugs anymore, I am where I need to be and I know what I need to do. So if you are worried that I'm going to become an ayahuasca junkie or something, you can rest assured, and you can tell my parents that too.

The patient further related that he felt "in perfect health," stating that he was sleeping well, eating a healthy diet, reading a lot, learning how to meditate, and contemplating joining a not-for-profit venture aimed at promoting ecological awareness and sustainable living. He denied psychotic symptoms, including auditory hallucinations or delusions; depressive and manic symptoms; anxiety symptoms; and suicidality or homicidality. His mental status examination was remarkable only for rapid but interruptible speech. A subsequent interview with his parents confirmed the absence of manic, psychotic, or other psychiatric signs and symptoms.

Discussion

In forming a clinical impression and treatment strategy for an individual using hallucinogens, there are three main questions to consider: 1) Does the individual have any vulnerabilities? 2) What hallucinogens were used, and were the circumstances of their use? 3) What are the acute and persistent effects of the hallucinogen? We investigate each of these questions in turn, considering them first in a general sense and then applying them to the case of Oswald.

Does the Individual Have Any Vulnerabilities?

Hallucinogen use can be problematic in individuals with certain psychiatric vulnerabilities or in those undergoing substantial stress. Hallucinogenic effects can present significant mental strain even in healthy, resilient, and stable individuals. As such, individuals already beleaguered by various stressors may be more likely to respond adversely to these effects or to experience a persistent reduction in stress tolerance following a distressing hallucinogenic experience. Similarly, individuals with poorly managed and destabilizing psychiatric or personality disorders, such as someone with active suicidality in the setting of a depressive illness, may further decompensate while experiencing hallucinogenic effects. It is also believed that hallucinogens may precipitate psychosis or persistently worsen psychotic symptoms in individuals with either a diathesis for psychosis or active psychosis, including those with Cluster A personality disorders. A history of problematic drug use likewise raises concern that the hallucinogen might be also used in an irresponsible or reckless manner. It is therefore important to assess for psychiatric disorders, family history, drug use history, and stress in individuals who are using hallucinogens.

The advice a health worker should unequivocally give to individuals with any of these vulnerabilities is to exercise great caution or avoid hallucinogens altogether. Even though emerging research suggests that subanesthetic ketamine might be effective for refractory depression and suicidality, it is not advisable for individuals with active psychiatric illness to take hallucinogens, including ketamine, recreationally or in an unsupervised setting given the possibility of clinical worsening. The role of the health worker when confronted with hallucinogen use in vulnerable individuals is to ascertain for clinical worsening and to provide psychoeducation, nonjudgmentally informing them of the serious risks they incur in continuing to use hallucinogens given their vulnerabilities. A patient who persists in using hallucinogens despite clear clinical worsening likely meets criteria for abuse and should be approached accordingly, with motivational interviewing the first strategy to be tried.

In the case of Oswald, no clear psychiatric vulnerability exists, including a diathesis for psychosis. Furthermore, his history of drug use, characteristic of many college students, does not raise immediate concern for abuse or dependence (although his history of binge drinking on weekends merits further exploration). However, he appears to be undergoing chronic stress in the context of several major life changes, including graduating from college, contemplating the next step in his life, and maintaining the individuation process even as he as returns to living at home with parents intolerant of his "alternative" life choices. The very same existential concerns that were creating stress, moreover, are those that led him to seek out the ayahuasca ceremony as a way of bringing some clarity to his situation.

As we discuss in the next section, looking to hallucinogens as a way of resolving conflicts or coping with difficulties may not always end on a positive or enlightened note. That the ceremony turned out well reflects Oswald's strengths: his intelligence, psychological resilience, and interest in ensuring that the hallucinogen was administered in a relatively responsible and guided setting. Whether it will ultimately lead to a persistent positive effect on Oswald's life, however, remains to be seen.

What Hallucinogens Were Used and What Were the Circumstances of Their Use?

The type of hallucinogen used can have important clinical implications. Certain hallucinogens are more likely to lead to problematic use patterns than are others. MDMA, nitrous oxide, and ketamine, for example, can produce dependence, and individuals using them regularly should be assessed and monitored closely for the emergence of a substance use disorder. Furthermore, MDMA carries life-threatening risks associated with elevated body temperature; patients should be evaluated for whether they engage in activities while intoxicated that might heighten this risk (such as dancing all night in a hot warehouse without proper hydration). Although not free of the risk for abuse, classical hallucinogens do not pose these same dangers. Classical hallucinogen use is followed by a generally 72-hour refractory period during which repeated doses of further drug fail to have an effect, thereby precluding the repeated and escalating administration that characterizes problematic use of other hallucinogens.

Another important source of clinical information is the context in which the hallucinogen use occurs, or what was designated earlier as the *set* and *setting*. As with many other substances, there are circumstances and environments in which the adverse effects of hallucinogens are more likely to be pronounced or are more likely to lead to impairment. Of particular concern is when hallucinogens are used in situations requiring a high level of functioning, such as at school or work, while caring for children, or while operating heavy machinery such as an automobile, given the propensity of hallucinogens to lead to acute deficiencies in behavioral control, attention, and decision making. Identifying that the hallucinogen use is repeatedly coupled with a particular behavior (such as using LSD whenever watching a film) is also worrying because it suggests that the drug use is becoming inseparable from a person's hobbies or pastimes. These repeated patterns of recreational intoxication may confer greater risk of developing problematic use. Psychoeducation and motivational interviewing techniques can be helpful in bringing attention to potential problems and possibly in effecting change.

The expectations, hopes, and desires that an individual brings to the hallucinogen experience are important to identify. Turning to hallucinogen use as a way of coping with stress can lead to the same risks that accompany using other substances for stress relief: developmental problems, particularly in regard to cultivating healthy ways of coping, and the entrenchment of poor coping skills. Furthermore, hallucinogen use in the context of high stress may lead, as mentioned earlier, to a greater likelihood of further distress and to decreased stress tolerance. Similarly, investing the hallucinogen experience with great existential importance, and hoping to find in the experience a far-reaching solution to life's problems, can also be problematic from a developmental perspective. The danger here is that a nuanced and healthy engagement with life's difficulties will be lost in the adoption of a simplistic narrative that constructs the hallucinogen experience into a dramatic transformation or turning point after which the usual problems and stressors of life cease to exist. Furthermore, this perspective may be associated with greater receptiveness on the part of the individual toward psychologically unhealthy world views, such as cult-based or fanatical religious belief.

Problematic expectations, if they come to clinical attention, should be addressed with psychotherapy. Skills training can also be helpful in identifying healthier ways of dealing with stress in those who consistently turn to hallucinogens for stress relief. Individuals who had hoped hallucinogen use would allow them to successfully navigate difficult life transitions may benefit from ongoing psychotherapy both to effectively incorporate the hallucinogenic experience into their lives and to provide support in effectively managing existential stress. Exploratory therapy may also be helpful in identifying psychodynamic reasons for why the hallucinogenic experience was sought as a stepping stone to a more fulfilling future.

The contexts in which Oswald used hallucinogens were similar over the course of college. He had used LSD twice at various parties without significant consequence, psilocybin once while hiking, and MDMA several times his junior year under unclear circumstances. His use of the three substances appears to have been guided by peer influence and perhaps by a desire for pleasure or novel sensations. The infrequent use of LSD and the clustered use of MDMA are common in young adults, and in the absence of clear problematic consequences, this use does not constitute a cause for alarm. His statement that he is "done with drugs" is open to interpretation, but it suggests that hallucinogen abuse or other use-related problems, never clearly issues for him anyway, are unlikely to emerge in the near future.

Oswald's recent use of ayahuasca merits greater discussion, particularly because it is the most proximal reason for his evaluation. It also represents a significant shift from previous hallucinogen use with regard to set and setting. Ayahuasca ceremonies are becoming increasingly more common in the United States, particularly in urban settings. They involve, as described by Oswald, a Western approximation of the shaman-supplicant relationship that is so central to certain preindustrial cultures. Furthermore, the ceremony revolves around the administration of ayahuasca (a plant-based brew whose primary constituents are DMT and a monoamine oxidase inhibitor, which serves to inhibit metabolism of the hallucinogen), as is the case with healing and religious practices in some Amazonian groups. The religious and "ancient" elements of the ceremony undoubtedly influenced the way in which Oswald experienced the effects of ayahuasca. Additionally, the shaman skillfully managed Oswald's expectations by priming him for a powerful spiritual journey with mystical readings and by maintaining a religious and ceremonial atmosphere throughout the experience. In this way, the set and setting were modified to facilitate the production of an experience of mystical importance.

Oswald also approached the ceremony with a different spirit than what had characterized his hallucinogen use previously. He was hopeful that the experience would guide him and resolve some of his existential confusions. This lack of direction had been occurring in the context of a difficult individuation process in which he was unable to assert himself in the midst of parental pressures: "playing the game so as to keep [them] off [his] back." He turned for insight and clarity to an illicit substance administered in a way antithetical to modern or Western norms of religious engagement, which underscores the rebellious function that the ayahuasca ceremony served for him. As had occurred in the 1960s for many young adults struggling to come into their own, the generational conflicts Oswald experienced vis-à-vis his parents were centered on hallucinogen use.

Clearly, Oswald may benefit from psychotherapy aimed at helping him to work through the difficulties he experiences with his parents and to understand why he turned to ayahuasca as a way to overcome these difficulties. These tensions with his parents, furthermore, are likely to intensify in the aftermath of the ayahuasca ceremony because he now feels a readiness to assert himself and make lifestyle and work choices with which his parents may not agree. Psychotherapy can assist Oswald in setting viable goals for himself, moving forward with his choices in a way that does not create unnecessary conflict with his parents and incorporating the hallucinogen experience into a life narrative that is healthy, resilient, and creative. The efficacy of the psychotherapy will depend, to some extent, on the willingness of Oswald to maintain openness and accept the emergence of new desires and goals that may not always be congruent with the self-identity he fashioned immediately after the ayahuasca ceremony (e.g., deciding to return to school for an MBA). This willingness to relinquish certain aspects of the experience, in turn, depends on the persistent effects of ayahuasca in the weeks and months ahead.

What Are the Acute and Persistent Effects of the Hallucinogen?

As mentioned previously, the most life threatening hallucinogen-related adverse event is MDMA-induced hyperthermia. This should be managed immediately with cooling and hydration. An intensive care consultation should also be obtained for subacute stabilization after acute cooling and hydration measures have been implemented.

A more common, and sometimes dangerous, source of hallucinogen-related acute distress is simple intoxication. In unprepared or unguided individuals, hallucinogens can occasionally lead to such high levels of distress that individuals may seek out medical help in the midst of the experience out of fear that they are going to die, become insane, or undergo some catastrophe. The acutely distressed individual will present to the emergency department, by ambulance or otherwise, and health workers will be confronted by a terrified, possibly incoherent, and behaviorally disorganized person who may not be able to properly recount what happened, including whether a hallucinogen was taken. Physiological signs of intoxication, such as dilated pupils, diaphoresis, and altered psychomotor status, may serve as clues in the absence of a clear history.

Hallucinogen-related distress can constitute a psychiatric emergency and may involve many of the usual features of acute decompensation, including poor engagement with health workers, agitation, aggression, elopement risk, or suicidality. A one-to-one sitter should therefore be assigned. Caution should be exercised, of course, and if the patient does not respond to supportive therapy, relaxation exercises, and redirection, a low dose of fast-acting benzodiazepine such as lorazepam should be sufficient to ameliorate distress. The medication should be offered by mouth initially, and if the medication is refused and pharmacological restraint is deemed necessary, then it should be provided intramuscularly.

Agitated patients are not identical, and the emergency measure of haloperidol 5 mg and lorazepam 2 mg intramuscularly, although effective for some agitated patients, is in excess of what is typically required for hallucinogen-related distress. Haloperidol should never be the first-line treatment for this presentation because it leads to serious risks without providing added benefit. Often, support, reassurance, and the administration of relaxation exercises (or a benzodiazepine) should suffice. Cases of agitation or aggression refractory to high-dose benzodiazepines, however, may benefit from haloperidol or another antipsychotic.

The persistent effects of hallucinogens can include the precipitation of psychosis, depression, or anxiety in vulnerable individuals or the exacerbation of psychiatric distress in patients with unstable mental illness. Psychiatric distress should be managed as it would be in other circumstances: worsening psychosis merits the initiation or higher doses of an antipsychotic, mania requires mood stabilization, and worsening anxiety and depressive symptoms require proper pharmacotherapy and psychotherapy. Clear cases of hallucinogen-induced depression or anxiety, however, should not be treated with pharmacotherapy immediately: watchful waiting, along with psychotherapy, is advised. If the depression or anxiety persists for more than 4 weeks after the hallucinogen use or if symptoms are so severe as to merit immediate clinical attention, then pharmacotherapy may be necessary.

The management of hallucinogen-induced psychosis is less clear-cut because it has not been properly studied. Furthermore, cases may be time limited and may resolve on their own without pharmacotherapy. It is currently impossible, however, to delineate at the outset between time-limited cases and those that might persist for some time. Expert opinion encourages the judicious use of antipsychotics for hallucinogen-induced psychosis, although the role of maintenance pharmacotherapy remains unclear.

As mentioned previously, a rare consequence of hallucinogen use is hallucinogen persisting perception disorder, or flashbacks. This differs from psychosis in that the effects are purely perceptual rather than involving cognition, behavior, or ideation. Unfortunately, there are no known treatments for this seldom encountered but distressing condition.

Persistent psychodynamic effects of hallucinogen use chiefly relate to the existential or psychological importance with which the experience has been invested. As discussed earlier, individuals may find in the experience insights that they feel will shape the rest of their lives. Such insights may be enriching or destabilizing, depending on the circumstances. Psychiatric attention (psychotherapy and cognitive restructuring) might be helpful for an individual tenaciously adhering to these insights even when they are leading to substantial distress, impairment, or isolation. It is important to emphasize that such ideation is different from delusional thinking. The phenomenon is perhaps most similar to the *overvalued idea* in which there is an unwillingness, but not inability, to entertain alternative perspectives or cast doubt on the cherished idea or insight. A man, for example, may decide while using LSD that he needs to hold various yoga poses for several hours a day in order to attain optimal health and insists on holding these poses even as this insistence compromises his ability to maintain a job or fulfill other obligations. The prevalence of such difficulties is unclear. On the other hand, emerging data suggest that hallucinogens, and psilocybin in particular, may lead to insights with persistent beneficial effects on the capacity for openness, compassion, and equanimity.

With regard to Oswald, we again focus on the ayahuasca ceremony. Oswald underwent a mystical experience of great value to him, which he wrote down in elaborate detail. His interest in sharing his narrative in full with the clinician further indicates how important the ceremony was to him and how helpful he continues to find the various insights he gained during the experience. Interestingly, however, he relates that these were insights he was bound to have anyway over the course of his life and that the ayahuasca simply served as a "door" for quickly accessing them. This suggests that he does not identify the insights as occasioned simply by ayahuasca and that they have a more general importance and, perhaps, origin beyond the hallucinogenic experience. This is reassuring with regard to Oswald's likelihood for further ayahuasca use; as Oswald tells the clinician, he feels he no longer "needs" ayahuasca or any other substance. However, his readiness to regard the insights as valid and not as drug-induced fantasies makes Oswald more likely to be persistently guided by his experience. This necessitates examining the impressions, decisions, and insights induced by the experience in order to ascertain how they might affect his life over time.

Fortunately, the insights Oswald reported are within the realm of a beneficial mystical experience and apparently do not involve any features that may lead to impairment or distress (such as a decision to hold yoga asanas for several hours a day). Oswald reports an increased capacity to appreciate the interconnectedness of nature, to acknowledge his mortality, to reverence the mystery and beauty of existence, and to recognize the importance of living a creative and fulfilling life in harmony with a higher power. These all suggest spiritual gains likely to lead to greater fulfillment and creativity (Miller and C'de Baca 2001).

Newfound mysticism and spirituality, however, should always raise concern for mania-related hyperreligiosity, particularly when they occur precipitously or in the setting of drug use. Oswald denied all symptoms of mania, and although his speech is rapid, he was neither pressured nor disorganized. His parents confirmed the absence of manic symptoms, an important element of his history given how frequently such symptoms are underreported. His greater interest in spirituality appears to be a genuine and enduring consequence of a powerful mystical experience occasioned by the ceremony.

As mentioned previously, Oswald is bound to face some challenges as he begins to carry out some of his decisions in a household historically unreceptive to alternative values. The conflict with his parents may be exacerbated, furthermore, by the tendency of Oswald to avoid productive dialogue with them. He was brought to the emergency department, after all, primarily because the family was having a difficult time understanding him and was assuming the worst. There is a clear role for psychotherapy and family therapy in managing these difficulties. These interventions may serve to assist Oswald in asserting himself and his goals in a way that engages, rather than alienates or confuses, his family. Psychotherapy can also provide support and an opportunity for self-reflection as he continues to shape his life in a way that is more satisfying for him.

Conclusions

The case of Oswald illustrates the clinical complexity of hallucinogen use. By methodically investigating the three main diagnostic questions, however, we were able to elucidate the clinical issues and formulate a strategy for their management. It became clear that Oswald does not have hallucinogen abuse or other use-related problems, but he may benefit from psychotherapy aimed at supporting his decisions and goals, exploring his existential difficulties, navigating his relationship with his family, and incorporating his prior hallucinogen use into a life narrative that is open, creative, and resilient.

Other cases of hallucinogen use, particularly if associated with impairment or psychiatric sequelae, may require more intensive psychiatric support, including motivational interviewing, pharmacotherapy, or inpatient stabilization. When overwhelmed with clinical detail, it can be helpful to return to the three main diagnostic questions. Assessing for a patient's vulnerabilities, the circumstances of hallucinogen use, and the acute and persistent effects of use can provide an important foundation for understanding whether and what type of clinical management is necessary.

Key Points

- Dependence is not typically seen with most hallucinogens, but common complications include abuse, intoxication-related distress, and clinical worsening of unstable psychiatric disorders.
- In formulating a clinical impression and treatment strategy, three main questions should be addressed:
  - Does the individual have any vulnerabilities that render hallucinogen use particularly risky?
  - What type(s) of hallucinogens are used, and what are the circumstances of use?
  - What are the acute and persistent effects of hallucinogen use?
- Supportive psychotherapy can help individuals manage both the immediate and enduring effects of hallucinogen use.

References

Bakalar J, Grinspoon L: Psychedelic Drugs Reconsidered, 3rd Edition. New York, Lindemith Center, 1997

Galanter M, Kleber HD (eds): The American Psychiatric Publishing Textbook of Substance Abuse Treatment, 4th Edition. Washington, DC, American Psychiatric Publishing, 2008

Griffiths RR, Richards WA, McCann U, et al: Psilocybin can occasion mystical-type experiences having substantial and sustained personal meaning and spiritual significance. Psychopharmacology (Berl) 187:268–283; discussion 284–292, 2006

Miller WR, C'de Baca J: Quantum Change: When Epiphanies and Sudden Insights Transform Ordinary Lives. New York, Guilford, 2001

Sadock BJ, Sadock VA, Ruiz P (eds): Kaplan and Sadock's Comprehensive Textbook of Psychiatry, Vol 1, 9th Edition. Philadelphia, PA, Lippincott Williams and Wilkins, 2009

Vollenweider FX, Kometer M: The neurobiology of psychedelic drugs: implications for the treatment of mood disorders. Nat Rev Neurosci 11:642–651, 2010

Questions

5.1 Possible neurobiological mechanisms of hallucinogenic effects include all of the following except

A. Serotonin release.
B. Kappa receptor antagonism.
C. Effects involving the endocannabinoid system.
D. Selective serotonin receptor agonism.
E. *N*-methyl-D-aspartate receptor antagonism.

The correct answer is B.

It is κ agonism, not antagonism, that leads to hallucinogenic effects. The other mechanisms have been implicated in the effects of various hallucinogens.

5.2 Which of the following is the most common adverse effect of psilocybin?

A. Overdose.
B. Dependence.
C. Abuse.
D. Acute distress.
E. Acute psychosis.

The correct answer is D.

The most common adverse effect of all hallucinogens is acute distress related to intoxication.

5.3 All of the following can be helpful in managing hallucinogen-related problems except

A. Psychotherapy for managing acute distress.
B. Benzodiazepines.
C. Motivational interviewing for abuse or problem use.
D. Naltrexone to ameliorate cravings for hallucinogens.
E. Haloperidol for hallucinogen-induced psychosis.

The correct answer is D.

Naltrexone has not been investigated as a treatment for hallucinogen-related cravings.

5.4 What vulnerability places individuals at greatest risk for problematic hallucinogen use?

A. Father with depression.
B. Personal history of hallucinogen-related distress.
C. Alcohol dependence.
D. Maternal uncle with schizophrenia.
E. Large academic workload.

The correct answer is C.

Alcohol dependence places individuals at risk for problematic hallucinogen use. Previous intoxication-related distress with hallucinogens does not predict subsequent experiences. A first-degree family history of psychosis, not of depression, places individuals at risk. Although stress may be a vulnerability, it is relatively modest compared with alcohol dependence.

5.5 Which hallucinogen does not have a history of therapeutic or religious uses?

A. MDMA.
B. Psilocybin.
C. DMT.
D. Ketamine.
E. *Salvia divinorum.*
F. None of the above.

The correct answer is F.

All of the hallucinogens listed have been used in either therapeutic or religious settings.

CHAPTER 6

Inhalants

Just say N_2O!

Aykut Ozden, M.D.
Shaneel Shah, M.D.

INHALANT use is a widespread practice mainly among children and adolescents in developed and developing areas (Medina-Mona and Real 2008). The estimated risk of using inhalant drugs increased steadily among U.S. adolescents during the 1980s and early 1990s (Neumark et al. 1998). Results of the Monitoring the Future study indicated that in the 1990s, marijuana and inhalant drugs competed with each other as the first and second most commonly used substances among 12- to 17-year-olds in the United States, with inhalants being the most commonly abused illicit substance for several years (Johnston et al. 2013). The same study showed in 2012 that 11.8% of 8th graders had used inhalants in their lifetime, which is a significant number. Since the beginning of the 2000s, use of inhalants has remained fairly consistent, making it a significant health problem among adolescents. Inhalants are cheap, readily available even at home, and often legal to buy, so it is not surprising that they are abused by youngsters at alarming rates.

Inhalants are any gases or fumes that can be inhaled for the purpose of getting high. There are different ways of classifying these substances. On the basis of common profiles of pharmacological and behavioral effects, they can be classified into the following three categories (Balster 1998):

1. Volatile alkyl nitrites
2. Nitrous oxide (N_2O)
3. Volatile solvents, fuels, and anesthetics

The prototype volatile alkyl nitrite is amyl nitrite, which has been used medically in the past for treatment of angina. Abuse of nitrites began in the 1960s when ampules of amyl nitrites were "popped" open—hence the name "poppers"—and used for recreational purposes (Balster 1998). Nitrous oxide (N_2O), commonly known as laughing gas, is a widely used gaseous anesthetic. It is also found in whipped cream dispenser chargers and in aerosol whipped cream canisters sold for household use. Its reinforcing effects have been demonstrated in both animals and humans. N_2O acts on various neurotransmitter systems, including the opiate system and γ-aminobutyric acid, the latter of which is assumed to be mainly responsible for the abuse potential via the benzodiazepine receptor system (Balster 1998). Volatile solvents, fuels, and anesthetics are a chemically diverse group of inhalants. Solvents such as toluene and acetone are found in paint thinner, paint and polish removers, and correction fluid. Solvents are also used in spot removers, dry-cleaning fluids, and glues. Fuels can be found in propane lighters, pressurized fuel tanks, gasoline, and refrigerants (Konghom et al. 2010). These inhalants work differently and produce diverse behavioral effects.

Inhalation is typically achieved through sniffing, "bagging," or "huffing." *Sniffing* involves the inhalation of vapors directly from an open container or a heated pan. *Bagging* is inhalation of vapors from a plastic or paper bag, and *huffing* involves oral inhalation of vapors by holding a piece of cloth that has been soaked in the volatile substance against the nose and mouth. Abusers also spray aerosol compounds directly into the mouth. Recreational use tends to happen in groups and typically progresses from sniffing to huffing to bagging in order to increase the concentration of the inhalant and intensify the desired euphoria (Kurtzman et al. 2001).

Inhalants, as a group, are potentially toxic to many different vital organ systems, including the central nervous, cardiovascular, renal, and hepatic systems. The reader should refer to other sources for extensive reports on specific adverse effects on various systems, but a brief summary is presented in Table 6–1.

TABLE 6–1. Adverse effects of inhalants

Specific inhalant	Adverse effects
Central nervous system	
Toluene	Toluene-induced encephalopathy, seizures, coma, cognitive dysfunction, dementia, cerebellar damage
Glues and paints	Peripheral neuropathy in a stocking-glove distribution
Cardiovascular system	
Aerosols, gasoline, toluene, and benzene	Cardiac arrhythmias—sudden sniffing death syndrome
Nitrites and nitrates	Orthostatic hypotension and syncope
Renal system	
Toluene	Renal tubular acidosis, urinary calculi
Solvents	Glomerulonephritis
Pulmonary system	
Volatiles and hydrocarbons	Hypoxia, asphyxia
Hepatic system	
Chlorinated hydrocarbons	Toxic hepatitis, hepatic failure
Bone marrow	
Benzene	Bone marrow suppression, leukemia, lymphoma, aplastic anemia, multiple myeloma

Clinical Case

Brad is an athletic but short-statured 20-year-old single white college sophomore who came to his first session with his parents. It was a mixed decision for him. He agreed that he needed to see a psychiatrist because he had attention-deficit/hyperactivity disorder (ADHD) but disagreed with his parents, who made the appointment, that a psychiatrist could make him stop "nitrous."

He almost immediately said, "I am not going to stop it. It's harmless, kid stuff.... I did worse things." He went on to describe his problem focusing in school and how it was upsetting him and making him fall behind. He said that he stays sleepy during the day without psychostimulant medications, which he had not used in a long time. He had to repeat his first year in college, spending long hours studying and "missing out in life" because of not being able to focus. He probably could have continued, but his father intervened, saying, "Nothing worked. I don't think he has ADHD, or maybe he does, but hard to tell." Brad's mother added, "He was not bad until fifth grade; then his grades began to fall, teachers complained, and then in high school, he was totally out of control."

Brad's parents reported that starting sometime in middle school they had taken him to different psychiatrists, who gave him several psychostimulants, but he experienced side effects and thus had to stop after a while. His father also claimed that Brad "abused his Adderall," using more than given, but Brad yelled back, "It was not working, that's why!"

His father then added another twist: "He is paranoid." Brad smiled, held his head in both hands, and shook his head in disbelief. His father continued to report that lately Brad had been accusing them of having someone follow him and that he was in touch with someone who tells him the future. Brad, seemingly upset again, raised his voice one more time: "He does.... He even told me about this visit, the office, the furniture.... You don't have to believe me."

It was time to talk with Brad alone. He watched his parents leave and sighed. He reported that the only reason he had come was to get medication for his ADHD, "not about drugs or other stuff." When asked more about symptoms of inattention, Brad described difficulties at home and school that included making frequent mistakes, becoming bored and distracted easily, leaving tasks halfway through, being disorganized, and losing things often. He added this time that he would not use atomoxetine because he did not believe it worked and claimed it did not work in his girlfriend, who reportedly also had ADHD. When questioned about his substance use, he reluctantly reported that he had been using N_2O for several years, along with marijuana and occasionally "other stuff." He had used heroin once and did not like it. Cocaine was "an amazing drug...mental orgasm," but he could not afford it. He had used mushrooms "a lot in the past," and "some were good and some not." Regarding other substances, he said he "hated" alcohol, was "not into" benzos (benzodiazepines), and found lysergic acid diethylamide (LSD) to be a "wonderful drug, very profound but scary." He admitted to using LSD once a year. He smoked marijuana on and off during weekdays but used N_2O almost exclusively over the weekends. He named N_2O as his drug of choice.

Brad reported that he had first tried N_2O "through a balloon in high school a few years ago," and now he can inhale "tons of it without problems." He said he had last used it a few days ago, about 60 canisters of N_2O. He claimed that he would buy "whippits," which come as small canisters (see Figure 6–1) in a case that contained about 600 of them. It cost him less than $80 a case, so it was very affordable. He claimed that he and his girlfriend used it together with another couple, and over 3 days they would consume "thousands of" canisters at times. When questioned about how he could get such large amounts without getting in trouble, Brad laughed and said, "it is all legal."

He reported that he used a cracker to open the whippit and then used a balloon attached to it to catch the released N_2O. He denied ever using a tank but admitted that he had inhaled other substances, mostly household chemicals, on and off since age 13. He admitted to feeling high on N_2O and that it made him feel better about himself, "see the world differently," and "understand things better." He did not describe any symptoms that resembled any withdrawal state, but he said he had significant cravings. He also admitted having used much more than he had intended and spending more money than he used to spend, but he did not want to quit despite some knowledge of risks associated with use of N_2O. He had passed out on several occasions when he was inhaling N_2O and had hurt his head and body because of falls, but he had never sought medical

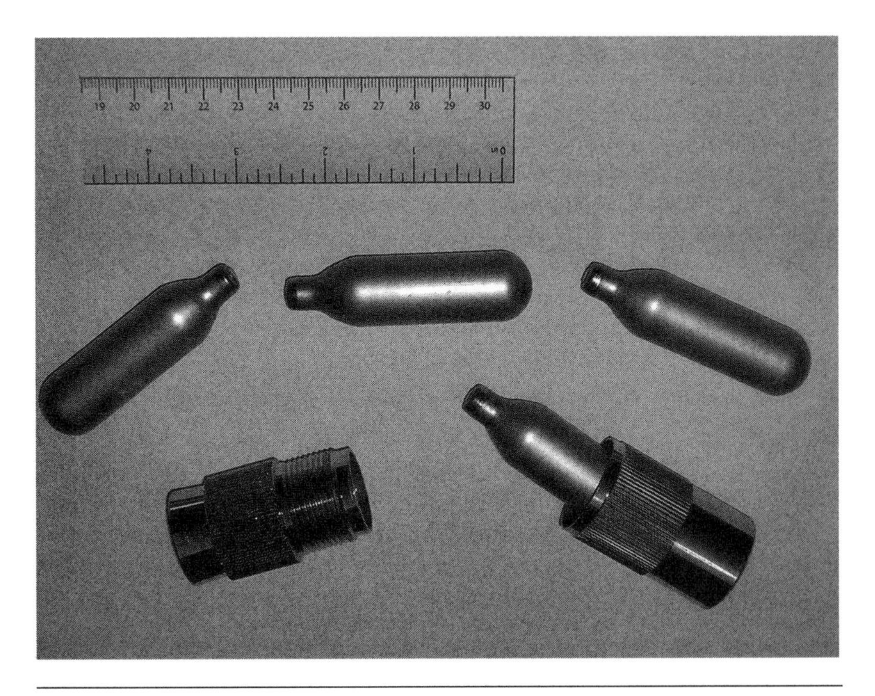

FIGURE 6–1. "Whippits" and an open nitrous oxide (N_2O) cracker.

care or gone to the emergency department. These incidents did not stop him from using N_2O.

Brad's parents later told me that he had become more forgetful and inattentive and was "not himself." They strongly believed that his "paranoia" started after he had begun using N_2O. They took him to several psychiatrists, who diagnosed him with cannabis and inhalant use disorders and ADHD. He had seen his primary care physician a few months earlier and been given a physical examination and laboratory tests, but they were not extensive. His parents were told his tests were normal. They had considered having him admitted to a rehabilitation center, but he always refused.

Brad had never had any psychiatric problems until recently, except for problems with his attention and hyperactivity. He had developed some oppositional behavior in middle school and had started to gravitate toward nonacademic friends. He would come home late and cut school, but he was never violent and never acted antisocially. He was able to finish high school with difficulty and got into a college, where his problems escalated and he had to repeat his freshman year. His parents blamed his increased drug use for his declining academic performance, whereas Brad believed it was due to not finding the right medication for his ADHD. He even accused his parents of giving him "fake medications" lately because the medications had no effect in him. He increased the dosages of his stimulants himself, which then caused his last psychiatrist to terminate his treatment. Brad denied abusing his stimulant medications and said he never felt high on them. He claimed he was very sleepy and inattentive without them, but a sleep study had been done in the past and did not reveal any problems.

Brad's early childhood was unremarkable, with normal development and no history of trauma or separation. He did not have any known medical problems, and in his family there were two cousins with ADHD and members with alcoholism on both sides but not in his parents.

On the basis of the reports of both Brad and his parents, the initial diagnoses were inhalant dependence, cannabis dependence, and ADHD. Because Brad's psychotic symptoms presented with escalating substance use, a diagnosis of substance-induced psychotic disorder was also made. He did not fulfill criteria for other psychotic symptoms and did not have any mood disorder. It was difficult to know which one was causing the psychotic symptoms, N_2O or cannabis, because he used both almost regularly in high doses and for a long time. However, his parents were certain that it was the former. They reported that he had increased his N_2O use over the past year, and his paranoid symptoms began and got worse during that time. He had not been taking any stimulant medication while he had his recent psychotic symptoms.

Because of the presence of significant psychiatric symptoms, ongoing heavy substance use, decreased functioning, and possible neurological problems, inpatient rehabilitation was recommended. The parents agreed, but Brad flat-out rejected the idea. He did, however, agree to return for another evaluation session. He also agreed to have more blood work performed and to consider seeing a neurologist. He again asked for a prescription of a stimulant, which was rejected because of his ongoing psychotic symptoms. In return, he refused to try low-dose risperidone, stating it was not needed because he was "not paranoid." Psychoeducation regarding the potential psychiatric and medical effects of N_2O and cannabis was provided, including the names of some Web sites for Brad to check on his own.

Brad returned alone to his second session a week later. He said he had not smoked marijuana since his previous session, for which he was praised, but he had used N_2O as before. He said he did not believe he could stop right away because it was something he liked to do with his girlfriend, and they were joined by one or two friends at times. He also repeated that he still did not believe N_2O would hurt him because nothing had happened even though he had been consuming a lot. It was obvious that he was in precontemplation phase for his N_2O use. He agreed to participate in therapy sessions but mostly because his parents were going to cut off his money if he did not. He said he would do the blood work soon but was not sure if he needed to see a neurologist. His Mini-Mental State Examination score was 26 out of 30, which revealed memory and attention problems and indicated further assessment, but he was trying to turn it into a power struggle; he would ask for something, and when his request was rejected, he refused to do something asked of him. Therefore, the decision was made to delay neurological examination even though it was indicated. The approach chosen was to try to increase Brad's motivation to seek treatment and decrease his consumption of N_2O in a nonconfrontational way. In the past Brad had left psychiatrists who were confrontational and who insisted on rehabilitation or mutual help groups.

Motivational interviewing and motivational enhancement therapy have been used successfully in similar patients with low motivation and high resistance. Some of the features of motivational interviewing are using empathy, avoiding confrontation, avoiding opposing patient resistance, and developing discrepancy between the patient's goals and current behavior. Over the next three sessions, Brad engaged in a discussion reviewing his life, goals, aspirations, and expectations and how his heavy consumption of N_2O fit into them. He reported a wish to be financially independent of his parents, finish college, and go to graduate school, with the goal of becoming a lawyer like his father. He also verbalized his girlfriend's role in his ongoing consumption of N_2O. His ADHD was confirmed, but he would not accept nonstimulant medications. Another discussion centered on the effects of N_2O on attention and other cognitive functions, with which he already had a problem.

Brad stopped insisting on getting a prescription for a psychostimulant; however, he failed to follow up on blood work or seeing a neurologist. His psychosis remained unchanged because he was still using N_2O and refusing any antipsychotic medication. He was not acting on any delusion but kept stating that his parents were having him followed occasionally and that his friend could still the future. Neither of these was challenged because to do so would make Brad more defensive. However, he agreed for the first time that these thoughts were confusing and were stressing him, and he admitted that he was "afraid" of his friend because of "his power." He also acknowledged for the first time that there may be *some* relation between his N_2O and cannabis use and these thoughts. It was an unexpectedly early breakthrough. I invited his parents to his next session, and they came, but he was not present. His parents reported that he had agreed to check into a rehabilitation center after "getting high one more time." His parents asked questions about his prognosis and what to do after rehabilitation.

Brad stayed in rehab for about 5 weeks, longer than usual, and was discharged to a substance abuse therapist who was working in the same town where he attended college. He was not referred to a psychiatrist because he was not receiving any psychotropic medications on discharge. In rehab, he continued to refuse any medications except those for ADHD, which were not prescribed. According to his parents, his psychotic symptoms all but disappeared while he was in rehab; however, "it took a while." His father said over the phone that Brad would still claim what he had said prior to rehab was all true, but he would not talk about those claims anymore or blame his parents. His laboratory results were within normal limits, but a neurological workup revealed mild neuropathy. He was given vitamin B_{12}, which reportedly helped. Another positive improvement was that he had broken up with his girlfriend, who was a heavy user.

Discussion

There is a dearth of evidence-based recommendations for the treatment of inhalant use disorder. A review done in 2010 (Konghom et al. 2010) did not find a single randomized controlled trial on inhalant abuse and dependence treatment. The same review found a randomized controlled trial that studied carbamazepine and haloperidol in patients with inhalant-induced psychosis, but the trial focused on the improvement of psychotic symptoms. Authors of the review postulated reasons for the lack of available evidence: inhalant users may not recognize inhalant-related problems and thus may not seek treatment; inhalant users tend to be polysubstance users; inhalant use disorder often goes unrecognized by clinicians; and most people with inhalant use disorder are youths in probation systems, which makes it difficult to conduct a trial. Other than the last one, these descriptors fit into Brad's case. He was in denial; his previous caregivers had focused on his ADHD rather than his inhalant and cannabis use; and he used multiple substances, with N_2O being the most desired.

Regardless of the lack of well-designed studies, the National Inhalant Prevention Coalition (www.inhalants.org) has the following guidelines for the treatment of inhalant use disorders (see Box 6–1):

1. A medical examination to assess for the medical complications just described should be performed.
2. The detoxification period can be much longer—several weeks—than for other substances because inhalants are stored in the fatty tissue and are released gradually, causing altered affect and cognitive changes.
3. Although neurological impairment is usually present with chronic inhalant abuse, it is important to distinguish acute intoxication (Box 6–2) from long-lasting adverse effects. Repeat neuropsychological testing may help to assess for improvement.
4. Comorbid substance use should be treated as well.
5. Treatment programs should be prepared to engage the inhalant abuser in an extended period of supportive care because the 28-day treatment stay may be too short to expect change.
6. Psychosocial treatments play an important role. Different psychosocial interventions include exploration of peer dynamics because peer pressure is often a crucial factor perpetuating use, involving families and providing drug education and parenting and social bonding skills training, and arranging intensive aftercare to reintegrate the person back into society.

These are also all valid points and were followed in the treatment of this patient. Brad clearly needed a higher level of care, which he refused, but with the help of motivational interviewing rather than a confrontational "intervention," he agreed. His family was included in his treatment because they were instrumental in his recovery. He did stay in rehab longer than usual, during which it was found that he indeed had neurological adverse effects from chronic heavy consumption of N_2O and received treatment. He had comorbid psychiatric (ADHD) and substance use (cannabis) disorders. Brad could not *just say no* because it was very hard for him to do that alone and he was not ready, but with therapy and guidance he chose to do so by going into treatment.

Box 6–1. DSM-5 Criteria for Inhalant Use Disorder

A. A problematic pattern of use of a hydrocarbon-based inhalant substance leading to clinically significant impairment or distress, as manifested by at least two of the following, occurring within a 12-month period:

1. The inhalant substance is often taken in larger amounts or over a longer period than was intended.
2. There is a persistent desire or unsuccessful efforts to cut down or control use of the inhalant substance.
3. A great deal of time is spent in activities necessary to obtain the inhalant substance, use it, or recover from its effects.
4. Craving, or a strong desire or urge to use the inhalant substance.
5. Recurrent use of the inhalant substance resulting in a failure to fulfill major role obligations at work, school, or home.
6. Continued use of the inhalant substance despite having persistent or recurrent social or interpersonal problems caused or exacerbated by the effects of its use.
7. Important social, occupational, or recreational activities are given up or reduced because of use of the inhalant substance.
8. Recurrent use of the inhalant substance in situations in which it is physically hazardous.
9. Use of the inhalant substance is continued despite knowledge of having a persistent or recurrent physical or psychological problem that is likely to have been caused or exacerbated by the substance.
10. Tolerance, as defined by either of the following:
    a. A need for markedly increased amounts of the inhalant substance to achieve intoxication or desired effect.
    b. A markedly diminished effect with continued use of the same amount of the inhalant substance.

Specify **the particular inhalant:** When possible, the particular substance involved should be named (e.g., "solvent use disorder").

Specify if:

In early remission: After full criteria for inhalant use disorder were previously met, none of the criteria for inhalant use disorder have been met for at least 3 months but for less than 12 months (with the exception that Criterion A4, "Craving, or a strong desire or urge to use the inhalant substance," may be met).

In sustained remission: After full criteria for inhalant use disorder were previously met, none of the criteria for inhalant use disorder have been met at any time during a period of 12 months or longer (with the exception that Criterion A4, "Craving, or a strong desire or urge to use the inhalant substance," may be met).

Specify if:

In a controlled environment: This additional specifier is used if the individual is in an environment where access to inhalant substances is restricted.

Coding based on current severity: Note for ICD-10-CM codes: If an inhalant intoxication or another inhalant-induced mental disorder is also present, do not use the codes below for inhalant use disorder. Instead, the comorbid inhalant use disorder is indicated in the 4th character of the inhalant-induced disorder code (see the coding note for inhalant intoxication or a specific inhalant-induced mental disorder). For example, if there is comorbid inhalant-induced depressive disorder and inhalant use disorder, only the inhalant-induced depressive disorder code is given, with the 4th character indicating whether the comorbid inhalant use disorder is mild, moderate, or severe: F18.14 for mild inhalant use disorder with inhalant-induced depressive disorder or F18.24 for a moderate or severe inhalant use disorder with inhalant-induced depressive disorder.

Specify current severity:

305.90 (F18.10) Mild: Presence of 2–3 symptoms.
304.60 (F18.20) Moderate: Presence of 4–5 symptoms.
304.60 (F18.20) Severe: Presence of 6 or more symptoms.

Source. Reprinted from the *Diagnostic and Statistical Manual of Mental Disorders,* 5th Edition, Washington, DC, American Psychiatric Association, 2013. Used with permission. Copyright © 2013 American Psychiatric Association.

Box 6–2. DSM-5 Criteria for Inhalant Intoxication

A. Recent intended or unintended short-term, high-dose exposure to inhalant substances, including volatile hydrocarbons such as toluene or gasoline.
B. Clinically significant problematic behavioral or psychological changes (e.g., belligerence, assaultiveness, apathy, impaired judgment) that developed during, or shortly after, exposure to inhalants.
C. Two (or more) of the following signs or symptoms developing during, or shortly after, inhalant use or exposure:
   1. Dizziness.
   2. Nystagmus.
   3. Incoordination.
   4. Slurred speech.
   5. Unsteady gait.
   6. Lethargy.
   7. Depressed reflexes.
   8. Psychomotor retardation.
   9. Tremor.
   10. Generalized muscle weakness.
   11. Blurred vision or diplopia.
   12. Stupor or coma.
   13. Euphoria.
D. The signs or symptoms are not attributable to another medical condition and are not better explained by another mental disorder, including intoxication with another substance.

Coding note: The ICD-9-CM code is **292.89.** The ICD-10-CM code depends on whether there is a comorbid inhalant use disorder. If a mild inhalant use disorder is comorbid, the ICD-10-CM code is **F18.129,** and if a moderate or severe inhalant use disorder is comorbid, the ICD-10-CM code is **F18.229.** If there is no comorbid inhalant use disorder, then the ICD-10-CM code is **F18.929.**

Source. Reprinted from the *Diagnostic and Statistical Manual of Mental Disorders,* 5th Edition, Washington, DC, American Psychiatric Association, 2013. Used with permission. Copyright © 2013 American Psychiatric Association.

Key Points

- Inhalant use is widespread among children and adolescents, and it is important that clinicians specifically inquire about it when asking about other drug use.
- Adverse effects vary and can involve multiple organ systems, leading to different clinical presentations.
- Inhalants can stay in the system for a few weeks, especially if used chronically, which makes it important to distinguish acute effects from long-term irreversible changes.

References

Balster RL: Neural basis of inhalant abuse. Drug Alcohol Depend 51:207–214, 1998

Johnston LD, O'Malley PM, Bachman JG, et al: Monitoring the Future: National Results on Adolescent Drug Use. Overview of Key Findings, 2012. Ann Arbor, MI, Institute for Social Research, University of Michigan, 2013

Konghom S, Verachai V, Srisurapanont M, et al: Treatment for inhalant dependence and abuse. Cochrane Database of Systematic Reviews 2010, Issue 12. Art. No.: CD007537. DOI: 10.1002/14651858.CD007537.pub2, 2010

Kurtzman TL, Otsuka KN, Wahl RA: Inhalant abuse by adolescents. J Adolesc Health 28:170–180, 2001

Medina-Mora ME, Real T: Epidemiology of inhalant use. Curr Opin Psychiatry 21:247–251, 2008

Neumark YD, Delva J, Anthony JC: The epidemiology of adolescent inhalant drug involvement. Arch Pediatr Adolesc Med 152:781–786, 1998

Questions

6.1 Matthew is a white 12-year-old boy who has always been good at his studies. However, his grades have dropped over the past 3 months, and he has become more isolative. His parents have noticed paint stains on his fingers and mouth. They have also noticed that on occasions his eyes have looked red and watery. What is the likely cause?

A. Cannabis use.
B. Inhalant drug use.
C. Conjunctivitis.
D. Relational problem with parents.

The correct answer is B.

Inhalant drug use is common among 12- to 17-year-old children. Dropping grades and isolative behavior point toward the possibility of drug use. Whereas cannabis use can cause injected eyes and "amotivational syndrome" leading to poor academic performance, paint stains on fingers and mouth indicate inhalant use of products such as spray paint or nail polish. Adverse cognitive effects of inhalant use can adversely affect academic performance.

6.2 While doing an emergency department rotation, you are asked to see a 15-year-old boy with asthma exacerbation. During history taking it becomes clear that his concentration is poor, and he seems confused and uncoordinated. You suspect central nervous system (CNS) involvement and do a neurological examination, which shows intentional tremors. Urine toxicology screening results come back negative. What is the likely diagnosis?

A. Panic attack.
B. CNS infection with cerebellar damage.
C. Inhalant intoxication.
D. Delirium tremens.

The correct answer is C.

Inhalant use can cause respiratory tract irritation leading to asthma exacerbation. It can also lead to cerebellar damage and dementia-like symptoms. Urine toxicology screening does not detect inhalants because they are removed from blood through the lungs. Panic attacks typically have a more acute course and do not lead to memory impairment. In delirium tremens, resting tremors are common along with other features.

6.3 Kylie is a 17-year-old girl who is brought to the emergency department by the emergency medical service, accompanied by her friends. Kylie is drowsy and has difficulty following commands. Vital signs indicate tachycardia. During brief conversation, she complains of nausea. Physical examination reveals rhinorrhea and arrhythmia. Friends report that they were at a party, and Kylie was "huffing" with other friends. Diagnosis of inhalant intoxication becomes clear. What should be your first step?

A. Send urine toxicology to screen for other drug use.
B. Call Kylie's parents and inform them about her use.
C. Stabilize Kylie's airway, breathing, and circulation (ABCs) because inhalant use can lead to sudden death.
D. Wait for Kylie to wake up to obtain further history.

The correct answer is C.

Inhalant use can be harmful to multiple organ systems and can lead to sudden death. Cardiac arrhythmia can cause what is known as sudden sniffing death syndrome. Drowsiness may indicate CNS involvement and possible encephalopathy. Securing the ABCs is the best first step.

6.4 Andrew, a 15-year-old boy, is brought to your clinic by his parents. Andrew was hospitalized at a substance use disorders clinic 2 weeks ago for using paint thinner. Always a bright student, he has been doing poorly in school and has had poor memory and concentration for the past month. His cognitive problems have persisted since his discharge from the unit. His parents are certain that Andrew is no longer using inhalants, but they remain worried about his intelligence and ask your opinion. What should you tell them?

A. His cognition may or may not improve depending on the extent of use, but it may take some time for him to regain his capacities.
B. Inhalant use can lead to dementia, and his symptoms will likely persist for his lifetime.
C. Inhalants typically stay in the body much longer than other drugs, and his cognition will improve in the next 6 weeks.
D. He will need more neurological examination and testing.
E. A and D

The correct answer is E.

Although inhalant use can cause cognitive dysfunction and dementia, it is important to differentiate acute intoxication from chronic impairment. Effects can last much longer with long-term inhalant use, and patients can remain impaired even months after stopping use. A repeat neuropsychological test and examination can help assess for improvement.

CHAPTER 7

Opioids

Finding the Off Switch

Glenn Occhiogrosso, M.D.
Susan D. Whitley, M.D.

OPIOID use disorder is a chronic relapsing disease (Box 7–1). As with all addictions, genetic and social factors contribute to vulnerability. Tolerance and withdrawal may develop quickly, resulting in rapid progression from use to physical dependence to addiction. Craving and withdrawal drive the cycle of continued use long after the euphoric effects of opioid receptor activation have diminished. Adverse effects of use include high-risk behaviors associated with obtaining and using the drug, and significant mortality is associated with opioid overdose. The current epidemic of opioid addiction in the United States has been driven by misuse of prescription opioids, while at the same time rates of heroin use have remained relatively constant. Regardless of the opioid of choice, successful treatment involves management of acute withdrawal (Box 7–2), provision of long-term therapeutic interventions including medication-assisted treatment, and identification and management of medical and psychiatric comorbidities. The Drug Addiction Treatment Act of 2000 and subsequent U.S. Food and Drug Administration (FDA) approval of buprenorphine for the treatment of opioid addiction have created a new framework for office-based treatment in which general psychiatrists and primary care providers can fill an unmet need and help engage new patients in successful treatment.

Box 7–1. DSM-5 Criteria for Opioid Use Disorder

A. A problematic pattern of opioid use leading to clinically significant impairment or distress, as manifested by at least two of the following, occurring within a 12-month period:

1. Opioids are often taken in larger amounts or over a longer period than was intended.
2. There is a persistent desire or unsuccessful efforts to cut down or control opioid use.
3. A great deal of time is spent in activities necessary to obtain the opioid, use the opioid, or recover from its effects.
4. Craving, or a strong desire or urge to use opioids.
5. Recurrent opioid use resulting in a failure to fulfill major role obligations at work, school, or home.
6. Continued opioid use despite having persistent or recurrent social or interpersonal problems caused or exacerbated by the effects of opioids.
7. Important social, occupational, or recreational activities are given up or reduced because of opioid use.
8. Recurrent opioid use in situations in which it is physically hazardous.
9. Continued opioid use despite knowledge of having a persistent or recurrent physical or psychological problem that is likely to have been caused or exacerbated by the substance.
10. Tolerance, as defined by either of the following:
    a. A need for markedly increased amounts of opioids to achieve intoxication or desired effect.
    b. A markedly diminished effect with continued use of the same amount of an opioid.

    Note: This criterion is not considered to be met for those taking opioids solely under appropriate medical supervision.
11. Withdrawal, as manifested by either of the following:
    a. The characteristic opioid withdrawal syndrome (refer to Criteria A and B of the criteria set for opioid withdrawal, DSM-5 pp. 547–548).
    b. Opioids (or a closely related substance) are taken to relieve or avoid withdrawal symptoms.

    Note: This criterion is not considered to be met for those individuals taking opioids solely under appropriate medical supervision.

Specify if:

In early remission: After full criteria for opioid use disorder were previously met, none of the criteria for opioid use disorder have been met for at least 3 months but for less than 12 months (with the exception that Criterion A4, "Craving, or a strong desire or urge to use opioids," may be met).

In sustained remission: After full criteria for opioid use disorder were previously met, none of the criteria for opioid use disorder have been met at any time during a period of 12 months or longer (with the exception that Criterion A4, "Craving, or a strong desire or urge to use opioids," may be met).

Specify if:

On maintenance therapy: This additional specifier is used if the individual is taking a prescribed agonist medication such as methadone or buprenorphine and none of the criteria for opioid use disorder have been met for that class of medication (except tolerance to, or withdrawal from, the agonist). This category also applies to those individuals being maintained on a partial agonist, an agonist/antagonist, or a full antagonist such as oral naltrexone or depot naltrexone.

In a controlled environment: This additional specifier is used if the individual is in an environment where access to opioids is restricted.

Coding based on current severity: Note for ICD-10-CM codes: If an opioid intoxication, opioid withdrawal, or another opioid-induced mental disorder is also present, do not use the codes below for opioid use disorder. Instead, the comorbid opioid use disorder is indicated in the 4th character of the opioid-induced disorder code (see the coding note for opioid intoxication, opioid withdrawal, or a specific opioid-induced mental disorder). For example, if there is comorbid opioid-induced depressive disorder and opioid use disorder, only the opioid-induced depressive disorder code is given, with the 4th character indicating whether the comorbid opioid use disorder is mild, moderate, or severe: F11.14 for mild opioid use disorder with opioid-induced depressive disorder or F11.24 for a moderate or severe opioid use disorder with opioid-induced depressive disorder.

Specify current severity:

305.50 (F11.10) Mild: Presence of 2–3 symptoms.
304.00 (F11.20) Moderate: Presence of 4–5 symptoms.
304.00 (F11.20) Severe: Presence of 6 or more symptoms.

Source. Reprinted from the *Diagnostic and Statistical Manual of Mental Disorders,* 5th Edition, Washington, DC, American Psychiatric Association, 2013. Used with permission. Copyright © 2013 American Psychiatric Association.

Box 7–2. DSM-5 Criteria for Opioid Withdrawal **292.0 (F11.23)**

A. Presence of either of the following:
   1. Cessation of (or reduction in) opioid use that has been heavy and prolonged (i.e., several weeks or longer).
   2. Administration of an opioid antagonist after a period of opioid use.

B. Three (or more) of the following developing within minutes to several days after Criterion A:
   1. Dysphoric mood.
   2. Nausea or vomiting.
   3. Muscle aches.
   4. Lacrimation or rhinorrhea.
   5. Pupillary dilation, piloerection, or sweating.
   6. Diarrhea.
   7. Yawning.
   8. Fever.
   9. Insomnia.

C. The signs or symptoms in Criterion B cause clinically significant distress or impairment in social, occupational, or other important areas of functioning.

D. The signs or symptoms are not attributable to another medical condition and are not better explained by another mental disorder, including intoxication or withdrawal from another substance.

Coding note: The ICD-9-CM code is 292.0. The ICD-10-CM code for opioid withdrawal is F11.23. Note that the ICD-10-CM code indicates the comorbid presence of a moderate or severe opioid use disorder, reflecting the fact that opioid withdrawal can only occur in the presence of a moderate or severe opioid use disorder. It is not permissible to code a comorbid mild opioid use disorder with opioid withdrawal.

Source. Reprinted from the *Diagnostic and Statistical Manual of Mental Disorders,* 5th Edition, Washington, DC, American Psychiatric Association, 2013. Used with permission. Copyright © 2013 American Psychiatric Association.

Clinical Case

Donna is a 37-year-old former exotic dancer who was admitted for the first time to inpatient detoxification treatment for opioid addiction. She decided to come into treatment after she fell asleep in the kitchen while home alone, waking up when she banged her head on the edge of her kitchen table. This made her remember when she was a child and watched her own mother do the same thing. She says, "I realized that I was a drug addict just like her, and I had to get help." She came to the hospital later the same night requesting admission. Prior to this admission, Donna had been using $300 worth of heroin intranasally on a daily basis. Her daily use had been steadily increasing in quantity for the past 6 months, but in the days immediately prior to admission she felt she had completely lost control of her use. By the time she decided to seek treatment, she had been using more than $500 a day for the previous 3 days without sleeping or eating.

Donna began using heroin 2 years prior to admission when she could no longer afford to buy enough prescription opioids on the street to satisfy her addiction. Donna's first exposure to opioids was at age 24 when she fell and injured her back while at work and was given a prescription for an opioid pain medication by her primary care physician. Donna discovered that when the pain from her injury resolved, she could not stop taking the medication because "it made [her] feel something real." Over the next 10 years, Donna had a steady income and was readily able to get prescription opioids from doctors provided she had the money to pay for them.

Donna was raised by her mother until she was 7 years old. Her mother was an intravenous heroin user throughout Donna's childhood, and Donna remembers seeing her mother inject heroin in front of her and finding used needles in the apartment they shared. Her mother often left her in the care of friends and relatives, one of whom chronically sexually abused Donna starting at age 4. Donna believes her mother knew about the abuse and "let it happen because it had happened to her." The abuse stopped when her mother surrendered custody of Donna to her parents when she was 7 years old. Donna then lived with her grandparents until she started working as an exotic dancer at age 20.

After her admission to the inpatient detoxification unit, Donna was given methadone as needed on the basis of her withdrawal symptoms. During her first night, she had increasingly severe opioid withdrawal symptoms, including vomiting, diarrhea, and diffuse body pain. These symptoms intensified through the night, and she was unable to sleep because of the physical discomfort. She received three doses of methadone for the withdrawal along with an antiemetic to control her vomiting. This treatment provided her with minimal relief. Through the night and into the next morning, she was agitated, anxious, and extremely irritable toward members of the staff. The staff on the unit described her as "difficult" and "needy."

The morning after admission, Donna first met with her treating doctor, who determined that the dose of methadone she had received overnight was clearly insufficient in the management of her withdrawal symptoms. She was so restless and uncomfortable during the initial interview that she could not sit still. She repeatedly got up from her chair and paced as she discussed her history and condition. She was emotionally labile as well, angry while talking about members of the staff and other patients as she described her treatment overnight, then sad and tearful while talking about her history and desperation to feel better quickly. Donna felt more comfortable after talking to the doctor because he gave her a detailed explanation of the treatment she would receive on the unit and how it would rapidly lessen her withdrawal symptoms, which would allow her to sleep better at night and help her regain her appetite.

During this initial encounter, Donna told the doctor about her history of treatment with psychotropic medications for depression and anxiety. She had taken antidepressants, including sertraline, bupropion, and venlafaxine; antipsychotics, including aripiprazole and quetiapine; and anxiolytics, including clonazepam, diazepam, and alprazolam. Donna reported that the only medications that had ever helped her were the anxiolytics. She also reported that she had been taking all of these medications while still using opioids at high levels.

Donna started her formal detoxification treatment with a tapering dose of methadone her second night on the unit. Her withdrawal symptoms remained quite prominent for the next 2 days, and she continued to require long sessions with the treating doctor to help ease her anxiety. Donna told the doctor that she had seriously considered signing herself out of treatment many times over the course of the first 2 days. She reported that the memory of her condition prior to admission and the reassurance he had given her were the things that helped her to stay. By the third day of treatment, the methadone taper had reduced her symptoms enough that Donna felt well enough to sleep through the night. The following day her appetite began to return, and she ate full meals for the first time since admission. Over the next 3 days Donna was much better able to think about what she wanted to do after leaving the detoxification service.

Her addiction counselor presented Donna with multiple options available for the next step in her recovery. She was offered a referral to an inpatient rehabilitation facility, to the hospital's outpatient methadone maintenance program, or buprenorphine induction on the unit with continued treatment in one of the hospital's outpatient rehabilitation programs. Donna discussed these options with the counselor and the doctor the following day. She was reluctant to spend more time as an inpatient, not wanting to spend too much time away from her daughter, but did not believe she was ready to remain abstinent at home without maintenance therapy. She declined referral to the methadone maintenance treatment program because she found the requirement of having to go to the clinic every day too restrictive. After some nervous deliberation, Donna decided to initiate buprenorphine while on the inpatient unit.

Donna underwent the buprenorphine induction over the final 2 days of her admission. She responded well to this treatment and was discharged home on buprenorphine 7 days after her admission.

Donna started treatment in outpatient rehabilitation a week after her discharge and simultaneously initiated treatment with a psychiatrist with whom the treatment program had an existing alliance. Over the course of the first month in treatment, she continued to have some mild withdrawal symptoms and strong cravings to use opioids. Her buprenorphine dose was increased twice, and her symptoms and cravings gradually resolved. Donna initially attended groups at the treatment program three times per week, followed by a gradual reduction in frequency. She engaged in individual therapy with her psychiatrist to begin to address some of the trauma she had experienced as a child. Her anxiety and affective instability dramatically improved, "as if someone flipped a switch in her brain." More than 1 year after her admission, Donna has remained abstinent from opioids and has returned to school to get her GED with the hope of going on to get a college degree as well.

Discussion

Donna clearly met the criteria for opioid use disorder, severe, and benefited from the inpatient stay to stabilize and make decisions about care that would have been difficult for her to achieve on an ambulatory basis. The treatment team initially recommended referral to an inpatient rehabilitation. Some members of the team interpreted Donna's reluctance to attend inpatient treatment as an indicator of low motivation for change, but her counselor and physician continued to explore barriers and offered alternatives that better matched her preferences. Donna was clearly a candidate for maintenance treatment on the basis of her long history of use and multiple unsuccessful treatment attempts. Her refusal to accept referral to methadone treatment could also be interpreted as "resistance," but the team continued to engage her in discussion of alternatives. This case demonstrates the importance of providing choices in treatment. Only when Donna felt listened to and in control of the decision process was she able to commit to a level of care that could be successful for her.

In addition to opioid addiction, Donna presented with psychiatric symptoms including anxiety, dysphoria, and affective instability. Although the treating physician recognized these as possible evidence of an underlying psychiatric disorder, he chose to focus on the management of opioid withdrawal and alliance building, with the hope of successfully engaging Donna in care. Diagnosis and management were deferred, with detailed handoff to the outpatient treatment program. In fact, many of Donna's symptoms resolved on stabilization of her buprenorphine dosage. This case highlights the importance of carefully assessing and addressing psychiatric comorbidity when treating opioid addiction and highlights the advantages of integrated behavioral health and addictions treatment.

Treatment Settings

Treatment planning for opioid addiction involves two major decisions: the treatment setting and the role of medications. In this section we present an overview of levels of care and a discussion of available medications for the treatment of opioid addiction. This knowledge should guide a clinician's recommendations; however, finding the right treatment is best accomplished in collaboration with the patient. Although expert consensus will agree that psychosocial treatments are an essential component of success, the efficacy of one treatment modality over another has been difficult to quantify. Choice of level of care must therefore be based in clinical guidelines but strongly guided by patient preference. Offering options and honoring a patient's priorities will serve to maintain autonomy, improve patient engagement, and increase the chance that the right combination of medication and therapy can be achieved. Only then can the off switch be found.

Medically managed withdrawal, also known as detoxification, involves control of acute withdrawal symptoms. Withdrawal can be managed on an inpatient or ambulatory basis using FDA-approved opioid agonists including methadone and buprenorphine. Agents providing symptomatic relief (e.g., clonidine, ibuprofen, and loperamide) can be useful adjuncts. This short-term treatment does not provide adequate time to stabilize and reset the brain's opioid system, which has grown accustomed to receiving a supply of exogenous opioids. The unsatisfied opioid receptors produce continued lower-level withdrawal symptoms and craving. However, a detoxification episode is often the first point of contact for individuals seeking treatment and provides a teachable moment. Interventions should be aimed at reducing risk related to use, providing education regarding aftercare options including medication-assisted treatment, and increasing motivation to change. The efficacy of "detox" is often hindered by failure to follow through with recommended aftercare and high relapse rates. The measure of successful detoxification should be not treatment completion but rather successful linkage to the next level of care.

Inpatient levels of care may be especially helpful for individuals with unstable housing, limited social supports, and/or comorbidities that might impact their ability to sustain abstinence. Beyond detoxification, inpatient rehabilitation—"the 28-day program"—may provide a needed period of stabilization before return to the community. Therapeutic communities provide structured residential treatment, with a typical length of stay of 12–24 months. Peer interactions and group processes are used to influence behavior toward the goal of learning and assimilating more effective social skills. Despite the popularity of these treatment modalities, there is limited evidence for their efficacy over any other modalities, and reimbursement for inpatient levels of care has become harder to obtain.

Outpatient treatment programs provide a combination of individual and group counseling that generally includes education, support, and cognitive-behavior interventions aimed at relapse prevention. Program participation can be titrated to meet patient needs, varying from 5 days per week to one visit per month. The availability of resources to address psychiatric and medical comorbidities will vary from program to program.

Peer organizations such as Narcotics Anonymous provide a valuable source of support for many individuals in recovery. Some use community groups as a primary modality, whereas others use them in conjunction with formal treatment programs. Participation in peer support can be complicated for individuals using medication-assisted treatment because stigma against use of medication may exist. Patients can be encouraged to seek out groups that are more accepting of medication use and to focus on their general experience with addiction and recovery rather than the specific approach to treatment they have selected. Groups that specifically support medication, such as Methadone Anonymous, are available in some communities. Clinicians can help facilitate successful connection to self-help by having conversations about potential barriers and checking in about attendance and progress.

Attitudes about and access to medication-assisted treatment must be considered when making treatment recommendations. Some individuals may prefer abstinence-based treatment. In addition to patient preference, factors supporting the choice of abstinence-based treatment may include shorter duration of addiction, lower levels of use, and lack of significant medical or psychiatric comorbidities. Treatment programs, inpatient or outpatient, may have a preference for abstinence-based treatment. With the increase in evidence and regulatory pressures, more treatment programs do support the use of medication-assisted treatments. Some will collaborate with an outside prescriber, and others have onsite medical staff. It is important to be aware of the policy of a given facility prior to initiating a referral. In general, clinical trials support the efficacy of medication-assisted treatment, with improved retention and outcomes compared with placebo. It therefore stands to reason that regardless of the treatment setting, medication should be considered for most patients.

Pharmacotherapy

Opioid antagonists have demonstrated efficacy in the management of opioid addiction. Patients must be opioid free before the first dose in order to avoid the risk of precipitated withdrawal. Efficacy of daily oral naltrexone (Revia) has been limited in the real world by poor compliance. Extended-release injectable naltrexone (Vivitrol), approved by the FDA in 2010 for treatment of opioid addiction, can be administered every 4 weeks, thus reducing concerns about compliance. Efficacy remains limited because of failure to reduce craving to use opioids.

Another role for opioid antagonists, of the short-acting variety, involves reducing opioid-related overdose deaths. Injectable naloxone (Narcan) has long been the mainstay of emergency medical responders for the reversal of opioid overdose. More recently, public health departments in some communities have explored the role of distributing overdose rescue kits including naloxone to peers and family members of individuals at risk for opioid overdose. Intranasal naloxone is not currently FDA approved for opioid overdose reversal but has been used safely and effectively in multiple settings. Individuals who relapse to use after completing inpatient treatment or on release from incarceration are at increased risk for overdose because their tolerance has been significantly lowered and they may resume use at previous levels. Education regarding overdose risk is an essential part of treatment, and naloxone distribution is a cost-effective intervention with the potential to save lives (Coffin and Sullivan 2013).

The most well studied medication-assisted treatment is agonist maintenance treatment. Methadone, a Schedule II long-acting synthetic opioid agonist, has been at the heart of this discussion since its approval for the treatment of opioid addiction in 1972. Maintenance treatment of opioid addiction using methadone has a long track record of safety and efficacy (Ball and Ross 1991). Treatment with an adequate blocking dose provides relief of withdrawal symptoms while blocking both the craving for opioids and the reinforcing effects of these drugs. While receiving the proper maintenance dose of methadone, patients function normally and can focus on social and vocational goals often left behind in the cycle of addiction. Maintenance for 6 months or more is generally needed to achieve stability, and patients with long addiction histories and multiple treatment attempts may come to view maintenance treatment as lifelong. Methadone maintenance treatment has been repeatedly demonstrated to improve such outcomes as retention in treatment, reduction in illicit opioid use, reduction in criminal activity, and improved health and quality of life.

Methadone maintenance treatment in the United States is subject to stringent regulatory oversight and takes place only in specialized treatment programs. Opioid treatment programs (OTPs), commonly referred to as methadone maintenance treatment programs, provide a combination of medication-assisted treatment and psychosocial supports subject to federal and state regulations that dictate many aspects of treatment. Eligibility, with some exceptions, requires that the individual be at least 18 years of age with a minimum 1-year history of opioid use disorder. Programs are open 6 or 7 days per week. Frequency of program visits and criteria for obtaining take-home doses of medication are also dictated by regulators. Colocated treatment for psychiatric and medical comorbidities may be offered and has been demonstrated to improve outcomes. Although many patients, especially early in treatment, can benefit from this high level of structure, stigma and the need for frequent attendance are commonly cited barriers to access. Despite demonstrated efficacy, most individuals with opioid addiction do not enter OTPs, so we must continue to explore alternative means to engage patients in treatments that support abstinence and recovery.

The Drug Addiction Treatment Act of 2000 (DATA 2000) opened new doors for opioid addiction treatment. In the context of a national epidemic of opioid addiction fueled by misuse of prescription opioids, Congress passed DATA 2000 to allow for expanded access to care outside of the OTP setting. Physicians who are addiction certified or complete an 8-hour training course can receive a waiver from the Drug Enforcement Administration to prescribe FDA-approved Schedule III or higher medications for the treatment of opioid addiction. The law limits the prescriber to treating 30 individuals at a time, with the opportunity to expand capacity to 100 patients after 1 year. Prescribers must have the capacity to refer for counseling services, but there is no requirement for onsite psychosocial services. Buprenorphine, FDA approved in 2002, is the first drug to meet the DATA 2000 criteria and can be prescribed from a physician's office for opioid addiction treatment, including detoxification and maintenance.

Buprenorphine is a partial opioid agonist with a high affinity for the μ opioid receptor. This unique pharmacological profile results in a lower risk of misuse and overdose compared with methadone. Adverse effects and drug-drug interactions are also generally less common. Buprenorphine formulated with naloxone (Suboxone) further reduces the potential for misuse and diversion because naloxone will result in precipitated withdrawal if injected.

Buprenorphine induction describes the initial phase of treatment during which a patient is transitioned from his or her opioid of abuse to a dose of buprenorphine that relieves withdrawal symptoms. In some cases buprenorphine induction will be carried out on an inpatient basis; however, many opioid-addicted individuals will present for treatment in outpatient settings. In most cases induction can be safely carried out on an ambulatory basis and can be an extremely effective and satisfying intervention for both patient and provider. Buprenorphine induction, however, carries unique challenges, and concerns about the logistics of induction have been cited as a leading reason for provider reluctance to adopt office-based treatment of opioid addiction (Netherland et al. 2009; Walley et al. 2008).

Potential complications of buprenorphine inductions include precipitated withdrawal, an acute worsening of symptoms after taking the first dose of buprenorphine. Precipitated withdrawal can occur if an individual who is physically dependent on opioids and has opioids (e.g., heroin, methadone, or oxycodone) occupying μ opioid receptors receives a dose of buprenorphine. Because of its high affinity for the μ opioid receptor, buprenorphine will displace the full agonist, resulting in an abrupt decrease in net agonist effect. This can be expected to occur within 30 minutes after the buprenorphine dose is administered. Although symptoms are usually mild and easily tolerated, this possibility remains a major focus of concern for providers and patients. Patients experiencing precipitated withdrawal can require additional time and resources, including phone calls, office visits, and, rarely, emergency department visits.

To avoid precipitated withdrawal, individuals with physical dependence on opioids must be in opioid withdrawal at the time that the first dose of buprenorphine is administered. In its clinical guidelines, the Center for Substance Abuse Treatment recommends the use of standardized instruments such as the Clinical Opioid Withdrawal Scale for the assessment of withdrawal (Center for Substance Abuse Treatment 2004). The guidelines also suggest that the risk of precipitated withdrawal can be minimized by reducing the dose of the opioid of abuse prior to initiating treatment, allowing sufficient time between the last dose of opioid of abuse and the first dose of buprenorphine, and starting treatment using a lower buprenorphine dose. Treatment guidelines further recommend that inductions occur in the office of a qualified physician who can assess for opioid withdrawal, gradually titrate buprenorphine doses, and monitor patients' responses to buprenorphine. Use of long-acting opioids such as methadone, use of benzodiazepines, and anxiety symptoms may be associated with increased risk for complicated induction (Whitley et al. 2010), whereas individuals who have previously used buprenorphine (whether illicitly or by prescription) appear less likely to experience complications.

In-person assessment of opioid withdrawal symptoms and observation of initial dosing remain the standard of care. Clinical experience and a growing body of literature support the feasibility and safety of allowing patients to initiate treatment at home (Cunningham et al. 2011; Gunderson et al. 2010). Patient education and ongoing communication are essential components of successful home inductions. Patient selection should include consideration of risk factors for complicated induction. Safety concerns including unstable housing, limited social supports, and unstable medical or psychiatric comorbidities argue in favor of observed induction. Very unstable or high-risk patients may be admitted to an inpatient service for induction.

Individuals seeking treatment for opioid addiction are at increased risk for medical comorbidities. Routine screening for common comorbidities, including HIV and viral hepatitis, is recommended. Likewise, individuals entering medical care should be assessed for opioid addiction. Clinicians providing treatment for chronic pain must be alert to red flags and risk factors for misuse of prescription opioids. Provision of care for medical conditions associated with opioid addiction should include routine screening for opioid addiction and interventions aimed at engagement in treatment. Several models of integrated care for HIV and opioid addiction using buprenorphine have demonstrated feasibility and the ability to improve both HIV and addiction treatment outcomes (Altice et al. 2011; Fiellin et al. 2011). Integration of medical care and addiction treatment has generally been shown to improve outcomes.

Psychiatric comorbidities are common among individuals with opioid addiction, particularly affective disorders, anxiety disorders, and personality disorders. It is difficult to separate substance-induced symptoms from underlying psychopathology, especially in early treatment. For example, anxiety is a prominent symptom of withdrawal, whereas dysphoria can be a result of dysregulation of the endogenous opioid system, and behaviors related to obtaining drugs (lying and stealing) can appear identical to symptoms of antisocial personality disorder. Some symptoms may improve as acute withdrawal subsides, whereas others will worsen as the opioids used to self-medicate are removed. Unraveling substance-induced symptoms from those of an underlying psychiatric disorder takes time and patience. Recovery is achieved only when both disorders are successfully addressed.

Regardless of the presence of a discrete co-occurring psychiatric diagnosis, trauma must be considered as a contributing factor. Trauma is associated with initiation of substance use and the development of addiction. Individuals with substance use disorders are more likely to report a lifetime history of trauma as compared with the general population, and substance use–related behaviors put individuals at increased risk for ongoing trauma. The effects of opioids may be particularly appealing to individuals looking to escape anxiety, feelings of emptiness, and other negative emotional states.

Given the high rates of psychiatric symptoms, poor coping skills, and the physical discomfort of withdrawal, it is not surprising that anger, ambivalence, and acting-out behaviors are common, especially during early treatment. Past negative experiences with treatment providers, history of incarceration, and difficulty forming trusting relationships are factors that impair ability to engage in treatment. Clinicians must remain attentive to their own frustration and avoid reacting in ways that can rupture the therapeutic alliance. This alliance is a critical ingredient for treatment success and can be difficult to achieve in this patient population. Integrating treatment for co-occurring disorders can improve engagement by increasing the individual's sense of safety and control, thus reducing emotional barriers to accessing care. Many individuals will be well served by allowing their treating psychiatrist to take the lead in managing addiction treatment.

An attractive model of chronic disease care is emerging in which some patients can be well managed by a generalist, whereas others are referred to specialty treatment settings (Figure 7–1). Individuals may receive methadone or buprenorphine in the highly structured OTP setting. Buprenorphine can be prescribed from the more flexible outpatient substance abuse treatment program setting. Office-based psychiatrists or medical doctors can provide buprenorphine and brief counseling in a more easily accessible setting where treatment for identified comorbidities is also available. Individuals can enter treatment through any of these doors and be transitioned from more intensive services to less intensive (or vice versa) as needed. This model is responsive to patient wishes and respectful of patient autonomy in a manner that can expand access to care and improve treatment outcomes.

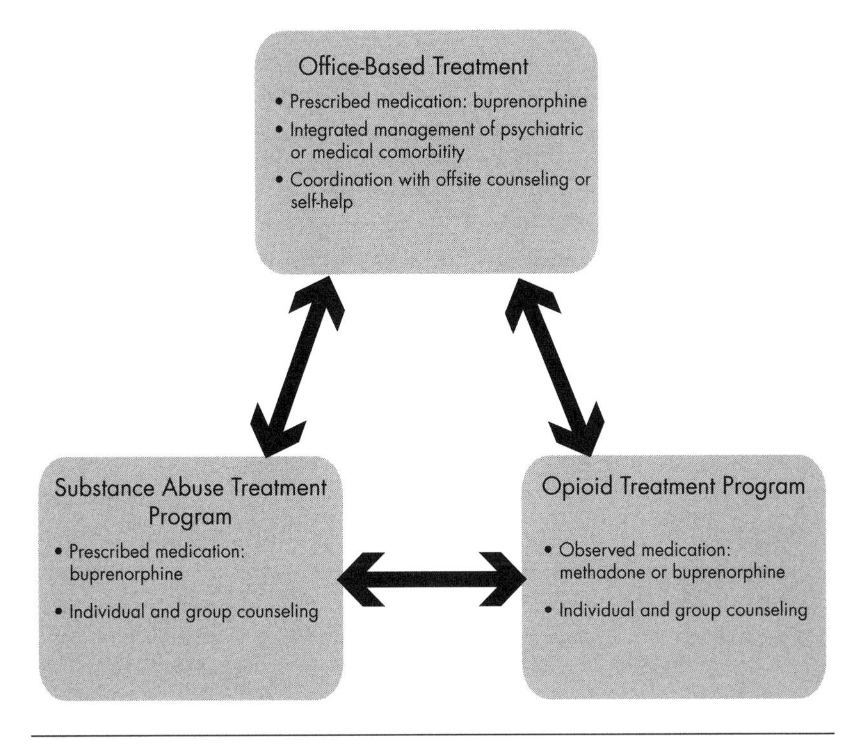

FIGURE 7–1. Model of chronic disease care for opioid use disorders.

Key Points

- Opioid use disorder is a chronic relapsing disease that requires a spectrum of care in which generalists and specialists share responsibility.
- "Detox" may provide a primary point of contact with the treatment system; however, it should be viewed not as an end point of treatment but rather as an opportunity to educate and increase motivation in longer-term treatment.
- Opioid addiction often occurs in the presence of a history of trauma and psychiatric comorbidity that enhances challenges of engaging patients in care. Providing choice and shared decision making around treatment planning can enhance motivation for change and improve engagement in treatment.

References

Altice FL, Bruce RD, Lucas GM, et al: HIV treatment outcomes among HIV-infected, opioid-dependent patients receiving buprenorphine/naloxone treatment within HIV clinical care settings: results from a multisite study. J Acquir Immune Defic Synd 56(suppl):S22–S32, 2011

Ball JC, Ross A: The Effectiveness of Methadone Maintenance Treatment. New York, Springer-Verlag, 1991

Center for Substance Abuse Treatment: Clinical Guidelines for the Use of Buprenorphine in the Treatment of Opioid Addiction: Treatment Improvement Protocol (TIP) Series 40. DHHS Publication No. (SMA) 04-3939. Rockville, MD, Substance Abuse and Mental Health Services Administration, 2004

Coffin PO, Sullivan SD: Cost-effectiveness of distributing naloxone to heroin users for lay overdose reversal. Ann Intern Med 158:1–9, 2013

Cunningham CO, Giovanniello A, Li X, et al: A comparison of buprenorphine induction strategies: patient-centered home-based inductions versus standard-of-care office-based inductions. J Subst Abuse Treat 40:349–356, 2011

Fiellin DA, Weiss L, Botsko M, et al: Drug treatment outcomes among HIV-infected opioid-dependent patients receiving buprenorphine/naloxone. J Acquir Immune Defic Synd 56(suppl):S33–S38, 2011

Gunderson EW, Wang XQ, Fiellin DA, et al: Unobserved versus observed office buprenorphine/naloxone induction: a pilot randomized clinical trial. Addict Behav 35:537–540, 2010

Netherland J, Botsko M, Egan JE, et al: Factors affecting willingness to provide buprenorphine treatment. J Subst Abuse Treat 36:244–251, 2009

Walley AY, Alperen JK, Cheng DM, et al: Office-based management of opioid dependence with buprenorphine: clinical practices and barriers. J Gen Intern Med 23:1393–1398, 2008

Whitley SD, Sohler NL, Kunins HV, et al: Factors associated with complicated buprenorphine inductions. J Subst Abuse Treat 39:51–57, 2010

Questions

7.1 Important factors to consider when planning treatment for opioid addiction include

A. Indications for medication-assisted treatment.
B. Availability of social supports such as housing and family.
C. Psychiatric comorbidities.
D. Patient preference.
E. All of the above.

The correct answer is E.

Although clinician knowledge of medication options and tools to guide selection of level of care will guide treatment recommendations, the best decisions are made when the voice and choice of the patient are included.

7.2 Methadone may be prescribed for the treatment of opioid addiction in which of the following settings?

A. Opioid treatment program or methadone maintenance treatment program.
B. Outpatient substance abuse treatment program.
C. Doctor's office.
D. All of the above.

The correct answer is A.

The use of methadone to treat opioid addiction is limited to licensed treatment programs subject to federal and state regulations that dictate many aspects of treatment.

7.3 Buprenorphine may be prescribed for the treatment of opioid addiction in which of the following settings?

A. Opioid treatment program or methadone maintenance treatment program.
B. Outpatient substance abuse treatment program.
C. Doctor's office.
D. All of the above.

The correct answer is D.

DATA 2000 allows for prescription of buprenorphine in multiple settings by physicians who receive a waiver from the Drug Enforcement Administration to prescribe FDA-approved Schedule III or higher medications for the treatment of opioid addiction.

7.4 Opioid overdose can be safely and legally reversed by which of the following?

A. Emergency medical provider administering intramuscular or intranasal naloxone.
B. Trained friend or family member administering intramuscular or intranasal naloxone.
C. Administering a sublingual dose of sublingual buprenorphine-naloxone.
D. Both A and B.
E. All of the above.

The correct answer is D.

Naloxone is used by emergency medical providers for the reversal of opioid overdose and, where available, can be administered by trained opioid overdose responders in the community. Although buprenorphine can displace other opioids, resulting in precipitated withdrawal, it will maintain some agonist activity and is not effective for reversal of opioid overdose. Naloxone has minimal sublingual bioavailability and will not assist in overdose reversal.

CHAPTER 8

Sedatives, Hypnotics, or Anxiolytics

Sleepless Nights and the Magic Pills

CLAUDIE H. JIMENEZ, M.D., M.S.
ABIGAIL J. HERRON, D.O.

SEDATIVE-HYPNOTICS are a class of medications that includes barbiturates, benzodiazepines, and, more recently, the "nonbenzodiazepine" hypnotics, comprising medications that act similarly to benzodiazepines for the treatment of insomnia. This last class, sometimes also known as "Z drugs" because their members include zaleplon, zolpidem, and eszopiclone, is the focus of the case presentation in this chapter.

Benzodiazepines are among the most widely prescribed medications in the world. Their approved therapeutic indications for mental health include anxiety, panic disorder, and insomnia, and they are also used in other areas of medicine for seizure disorders and muscle relaxation. They are highly effective in the treatment of these disorders but do carry a number of potential hazards, including physical dependence, overdose, and misuse and abuse.

The number of benzodiazepine-related hospital admissions nearly tripled between 1998 and 2008 (Substance Abuse and Mental Health Services Administration 2011). In 2009, sedative-hypnotics were involved in 363,000 emergency department visits, with zolpidem, a nonbenzodiazepine in the benzodiazepine receptor agonist class, involved in 29,000 of those cases, up from approximately 13,000 in 2004 (Substance Abuse and Mental Health Services Administration 2010).

The term *benzodiazepine receptor agonist hypnotics* is used to describe the classic benzodiazepines used for treatment of insomnia (such as diazepam) as well as the newer nonbenzodiazepine agents that became available beginning in the 1990s. These have become the primary pharmacological agents used for the treatment of insomnia over the past several decades (see Table 8–1). They share the same fundamental mechanism of action, although the newer nonbenzodiazepine medications have selective pharmacodynamic properties that may improve their safety and tolerability.

Benzodiazepines act centrally at the γ-aminobutyric acid A ($GABA_A$) receptor to increase the frequency of the chloride channel opening, enhancing the inhibitory effect of the GABA neurotransmitter. There are two types of $GABA_A$ receptors: Type I and Type II. Type I receptors are located in cortical and subcortical structures throughout the brain, and drugs with affinity for these receptors are hypothesized to produce sedation with little development of tolerance or dependence. Type II receptors are located in the limbic system, striatum, and spinal cord. These receptors are hypothesized to have a larger role in muscle relaxation and are more prone to dependence and tolerance development. The newer nonbenzodiazepine hypnotics have an affinity for Type I $GABA_A$ receptors.

TABLE 8–1. U.S. Food and Drug Administration–approved medications for insomnia

Medication	Brand name
Benzodiazepines acting at benzodiazepine GABA receptors	
Estazolam	ProSom
Flurazepam	Dalmane
Quazepam	Doral
Temazepam	Restoril
Triazolam	Halcion
Nonbenzodiazepines acting at benzodiazepine GABA receptors	
Eszopiclone	Lunesta
Zaleplon	Sonata
Zolpidem	Ambien
Zolpidem intermediate release	Intermezzo
Zolpidem extended release	Ambien CR
Melatonin receptor agonist	
Ramelteon	Rozerem

Chronic use of benzodiazepines can result in the development of physiological dependence, defined by the presence of tolerance and withdrawal symptoms (Boxes 8–1 and 8–2). *Tolerance* is present when escalating amounts of a substance are needed to maintain the desired (or therapeutic effect) or when diminished effects are seen with a constant dosage. *Withdrawal* is the presence of withdrawal symptoms when the drug is absent and is relieved by taking the drug or a similar substance.

The timeline for development of withdrawal symptoms depends on the duration of the drug use. Benzodiazepines vary widely in their half-life from a few hours to more than a day. Early symptoms of benzodiazepine withdrawal include anxiety, restlessness, and agitation and can progress to include abdominal cramps, increased heart rate, hypertension, hyperreflexia, tremor, insomnia, and seizures. This withdrawal syndrome can be life threatening. Individuals who have developed physiological dependence require medically supervised detoxification in order to safely discontinue their medications (American Society of Addiction Medicine 1999).

Despite a reduction in prescribing of benzodiazepines for insomnia, overall use of sedative-hypnotics remains high because of the frequent use of the non-benzodiazepine members of the class, which are now the most commonly prescribed hypnotic agents worldwide. Although these medications are sometimes considered safer than the traditional benzodiazepine agents, this remains controversial, and they are certainly not used without risks. These risks include adverse cognitive effects (such as memory loss), psychomotor effects (such as falls, fractures, and road traffic crashes), daytime fatigue, tolerance, addiction, and excess mortality.

Sedative-hypnotics are increasingly prescribed to the elderly population for the treatment of insomnia (McCall 2004). Although lower dosages of these medications are recommended for elderly patients, a proportion of patients misuse and abuse them, sometimes taking many times the recommended dosage. Side effects include central nervous system depression, abnormal thinking and behavioral changes, and anaphylactic reactions. Worsening of depression symptoms has also been reported. Unfortunately, substance misuse and dependence frequently go undiagnosed in this population. This may have a significant negative impact on medical comorbidities, cognitive impairment, and medication interactions. Medication misuse in the elderly is expected to increase. However, there is little research investigating the misuse of hypnotics in the elderly population.

Box 8–1. DSM-5 Criteria for Sedative, Hypnotic, or Anxiolytic Use Disorder

A. A problematic pattern of sedative, hypnotic, or anxiolytic use leading to clinically significant impairment or distress, as manifested by at least two of the following, occurring within a 12-month period:

1. Sedatives, hypnotics, or anxiolytics are often taken in larger amounts or over a longer period than was intended.
2. There is a persistent desire or unsuccessful efforts to cut down or control sedative, hypnotic, or anxiolytic use.
3. A great deal of time is spent in activities necessary to obtain the sedative, hypnotic, or anxiolytic; use the sedative, hypnotic, or anxiolytic; or recover from its effects.
4. Craving, or a strong desire or urge to use the sedative, hypnotic, or anxiolytic.
5. Recurrent sedative, hypnotic, or anxiolytic use resulting in a failure to fulfill major role obligations at work, school, or home (e.g., repeated absences from work or poor work performance related to sedative, hypnotic, or anxiolytic use; sedative-, hypnotic-, or anxiolytic-related absences, suspensions, or expulsions from school; neglect of children or household).
6. Continued sedative, hypnotic, or anxiolytic use despite having persistent or recurrent social or interpersonal problems caused or exacerbated by the effects of sedatives, hypnotics, or anxiolytics (e.g., arguments with a spouse about consequences of intoxication; physical fights).
7. Important social, occupational, or recreational activities are given up or reduced because of sedative, hypnotic, or anxiolytic use.
8. Recurrent sedative, hypnotic, or anxiolytic use in situations in which it is physically hazardous (e.g., driving an automobile or operating a machine when impaired by sedative, hypnotic, or anxiolytic use).
9. Sedative, hypnotic, or anxiolytic use is continued despite knowledge of having a persistent or recurrent physical or psychological problem that is likely to have been caused or exacerbated by the sedative, hypnotic, or anxiolytic.
10. Tolerance, as defined by either of the following:
    a. A need for markedly increased amounts of the sedative, hypnotic, or anxiolytic to achieve intoxication or desired effect.
    b. A markedly diminished effect with continued use of the same amount of the sedative, hypnotic, or anxiolytic.

    Note: This criterion is not considered to be met for individuals taking sedatives, hypnotics, or anxiolytics under medical supervision.
11. Withdrawal, as manifested by either of the following:
    a. The characteristic withdrawal syndrome for sedatives, hypnotics, or anxiolytics (refer to Criteria A and B of the criteria set for sedative, hypnotic, or anxiolytic withdrawal, DSM-5 pp. 557–558).

b. Sedatives, hypnotics, or anxiolytics (or a closely related substance, such as alcohol) are taken to relieve or avoid withdrawal symptoms.

Note: This criterion is not considered to be met for individuals taking sedatives, hypnotics, or anxiolytics under medical supervision.

Specify if:

In early remission: After full criteria for sedative, hypnotic, or anxiolytic use disorder were previously met, none of the criteria for sedative, hypnotic, or anxiolytic use disorder have been met for at least 3 months but for less than 12 months (with the exception that Criterion A4, "Craving, or a strong desire or urge to use the sedative, hypnotic, or anxiolytic," may be met).

In sustained remission: After full criteria for sedative, hypnotic, or anxiolytic use disorder were previously met, none of the criteria for sedative, hypnotic, or anxiolytic use disorder have been met at any time during a period of 12 months or longer (with the exception that Criterion A4, "Craving, or a strong desire or urge to use the sedative, hypnotic, or anxiolytic," may be met).

Specify if:

In a controlled environment: This additional specifier is used if the individual is in an environment where access to sedatives, hypnotics, or anxiolytics is restricted.

Coding based on current severity: Note for ICD-10-CM codes: If a sedative, hypnotic, or anxiolytic intoxication; sedative, hypnotic, or anxiolytic withdrawal; or another sedative-, hypnotic-, or anxiolytic-induced mental disorder is also present, do not use the codes below for sedative, hypnotic, or anxiolytic use disorder. Instead the comorbid sedative, hypnotic, or anxiolytic use disorder is indicated in the 4th character of the sedative-, hypnotic-, or anxiolytic-induced disorder (see the coding note for sedative, hypnotic, or anxiolytic intoxication; sedative, hypnotic, or anxiolytic withdrawal; or specific sedative-, hypnotic-, or anxiolytic-induced mental disorder). For example, if there is comorbid sedative-, hypnotic-, or anxiolytic-induced depressive disorder and sedative, hypnotic, or anxiolytic use disorder, only the sedative-, hypnotic-, or anxiolytic-induced depressive disorder code is given with the 4th character indicating whether the comorbid sedative, hypnotic, or anxiolytic use disorder is mild, moderate, or severe: F13.14 for mild sedative, hypnotic, or anxiolytic use disorder with sedative-, hypnotic-, or anxiolytic-induced depressive disorder or F13.24 for a moderate or severe sedative, hypnotic, or anxiolytic use disorder with sedative-, hypnotic-, or anxiolytic-induced depressive disorder.

Specify current severity:

305.40 (F13.10) Mild: Presence of 2–3 symptoms.
304.10 (F13.20) Moderate: Presence of 4–5 symptoms.
304.10 (F13.20) Severe: Presence of 6 or more symptoms.

Source. Reprinted from the *Diagnostic and Statistical Manual of Mental Disorders,* 5th Edition, Washington, DC, American Psychiatric Association, 2013. Used with permission. Copyright © 2013 American Psychiatric Association.

Box 8–2. DSM-5 Criteria for Sedative, Hypnotic, or Anxiolytic Withdrawal

A. Cessation of (or reduction in) sedative, hypnotic, or anxiolytic use that has been prolonged.
B. Two (or more) of the following, developing within several hours to a few days after the cessation of (or reduction in) sedative, hypnotic, or anxiolytic use described in Criterion A:
   1. Autonomic hyperactivity (e.g., sweating or pulse rate greater than 100 bpm).
   2. Hand tremor.
   3. Insomnia.
   4. Nausea or vomiting.
   5. Transient visual, tactile, or auditory hallucinations or illusions.
   6. Psychomotor agitation.
   7. Anxiety.
   8. Grand mal seizures.
C. The signs or symptoms in Criterion B cause clinically significant distress or impairment in social, occupational, or other important areas of functioning.
D. The signs or symptoms are not attributable to another medical condition and are not better explained by another mental disorder, including intoxication or withdrawal from another substance.

Specify if:

With perceptual disturbances: This specifier may be noted when hallucinations with intact reality testing or auditory, visual, or tactile illusions occur in the absence of a delirium.

Coding note: The ICD-9-CM code is **292.0.** The ICD-10-CM code for sedative, hypnotic, or anxiolytic withdrawal depends on whether or not there is a comorbid moderate or severe sedative, hypnotic, or anxiolytic use disorder and whether or not there are perceptual disturbances. For sedative, hypnotic, or anxiolytic withdrawal without perceptual disturbances, the ICD-10-CM code is **F13.239.** For sedative, hypnotic, or anxiolytic withdrawal with perceptual disturbances, the ICD-10-CM code is **F13.232.** Note that the ICD-10-CM codes indicate the comorbid presence of a moderate or severe sedative, hypnotic, or anxiolytic use disorder, reflecting the fact that sedative, hypnotic, or anxiolytic withdrawal can only occur in the presence of a moderate or severe sedative, hypnotic, or anxiolytic use disorder. It is not permissible to code a comorbid mild sedative, hypnotic, or anxiolytic use disorder with sedative, hypnotic, or anxiolytic withdrawal.

Source. Reprinted from the *Diagnostic and Statistical Manual of Mental Disorders,* 5th Edition, Washington, DC, American Psychiatric Association, 2013. Used with permission. Copyright © 2013 American Psychiatric Association.

The following case illustrates the impact of the use and misuse of a hypnotic agent in an elderly patient.

Clinical Case

Lily is a healthy 66-year-old retired teacher who takes levothyroxine (Synthroid) for hypothyroidism and has no previous history of alcohol or substance use disorders. She reported that she became "lonely and depressed" after she retired at age 65. Despite a large network of friends, she felt isolated at times because she had no close family of her own, and she missed the built-in socialization of the workplace. She had begun to withdraw socially, and although she had always "been a worrier," she now found herself with nearly constant anxiety. She began to lie awake at night wondering about the meaning of her life, worrying that she would "die alone" and that no one would remember her when she passed away. This situation began to recur nightly, causing insomnia, so she went to her primary care physician for help. She had no previous history of depression or anxiety and had no current or past suicidal ideation. Her physician prescribed a series of medications, starting with selective serotonin reuptake inhibitors (SSRIs) and later sedative-hypnotics, including short- and long-acting benzodiazepines and zolpidem. Each new medication initially helped her to sleep, but she found that the effect dissipated after a few days.

Lily's chronic lack of sleep led to daytime sedation and caused her to further withdraw from social activities because she felt too fatigued to participate. She began to increase the amount of medication she was taking without her physician's knowledge and repeatedly ran out of her prescriptions before they were to be renewed. She started seeing several physicians to obtain her medications. After 6 months, she was taking up to 3 mg of alprazolam and 100 mg of zolpidem daily. Her use was no longer restricted to insomnia, and she would often take 10 mg of zolpidem on waking in the morning. Lily was easily disoriented and reported walking her apartment hallways at night with no recollection of the events. On a number of occasions, she experienced hallucinations and ran up and down the hall in her apartment building yelling that there were intruders chasing her. Her neighbors called the police, and a mobile crisis team intervened on several occasions. Lily presented for substance abuse treatment when she was in danger of being evicted from her apartment because of this behavior.

In spite of requiring large amounts of medication to induce sleep and facing the prospect of losing her apartment, Lily initially insisted that she was not dependent on these medications but simply needed something to help her sleep. She acknowledged that she was taking too much and that the medications she was taking "were addictive." On initial evaluation, she denied symptoms of major depression or suicidal ideation but reported severe overwhelming anxiety regarding her insomnia. She described her nightly routine of falling asleep on the couch to a specific television show. If she was not asleep by the end of the show, she would take medication. If the medication did not make her drowsy shortly after taking it, she would take more medication until she slept. She began to have nights in which she did not sleep at all even though she took many times the recommended amounts of medication.

Lily completed a 5-day inpatient detoxification, during which time she was removed from all benzodiazepines and benzodiazepine receptor agonists. She then entered outpatient treatment, where she continued to report insomnia and significant anxiety related to her sleep. She was attending group therapy twice a week and individual counseling twice a month and was seeing an addiction medicine specialist weekly for her pharmacological management.

Amitriptyline, a tricyclic antidepressant (TCA) also used for the treatment of anxiety disorders, was started. Given Lily's past history of overusing medication and the risk of overdose with TCAs, she was given extensive education about the proper use of the medication and its risks and was also asked to bring her medication bottle to each visit for pill counts.

Early into treatment, Lily took a "handful" of "leftover" zolpidem pills when she could not sleep one night. They proved ineffective, resulting only in increased anxiety. She told her counselor and physician the next day and agreed to discard all old medication. From that time, she complied with her medication regimen and reported some improvement in her sleeping pattern over 2 weeks but still complained of anxiety related to her fears that she might be unable to sleep. Gabapentin 300 mg at bedtime was added to her regimen. We reviewed proper sleep hygiene practice and realistic sleep patterns, including sleep patterns of patients her age, and suggested that her ability to sleep "normally" would return in a few months. Even though Lily was very polite in receiving the information about sleep hygiene, she insisted that sleep hygiene would never work for her and, in fact, never tried any of the recommendations for the duration of her treatment. However, she did find that knowing that it would take time for her insomnia to resolve alleviated her anxiety.

Over the next few weeks, Lily's insomnia improved, and she started reengaging with her circle of friends, including meeting them for lunch dates and at the park. Lily also began taking up activities that she previously had given up because she had "felt too tired" to participate in them, such as going to the pool. Her visits with the physician were decreased to monthly visits.

After 3 months, Lily's sleep pattern returned to normal and the gabapentin was discontinued. Lily continued to participate in intensive outpatient treatment and continued socializing with her friends. She did have one night when she did not sleep and came into the office very anxious, stating, "It's starting again." We reviewed sleep hygiene recommendations, and I reassured her that the pattern would not repeat every night (even if it happened again that night). She slept much better (not all night) and felt less anxious. The next night she returned to her normal sleep pattern. After 6 months, Lily continued to sleep well, and the amitriptyline was decreased to 25 mg at bedtime. After 7 months, she continued to sleep well, was socially active, and later graduated from the outpatient substance abuse program.

Discussion

Lily initially presented with a complaint common among older adults: insomnia. She also reported a lifelong pattern of worry, which worsened significantly after her retirement and ultimately was focused on her insomnia. Lily's anxiety was both a cause and symptom of her insomnia and was ultimately relieved when her insomnia was treated. Lily illustrates an example in which benzodiazepines and hypnotics were used to manage insomnia and the patient ultimately wound up misusing the medication. In hindsight, Lily was at risk to misuse her medication. Factors associated with drug abuse in older adults include female gender, social isolation, history of substance abuse, history of mental illness (in her case perhaps mild anxiety), and medical exposure to prescription drugs with abuse potential. Lily reported being anxious and depressed over her life situation and experienced insomnia because of this. She was socially isolating from her friends when she was prescribed medications for sleep (American Geriatric Society 2012).

More than half of the elderly population has some chronic form of sleep disruption that may precipitate falls or aggravate other medical conditions. The use of sedative-hypnotics to treat insomnia in this group is increasing. Nonmedical use of prescription drugs among older women has dramatically increased (Bogunovic 2012). Commonly prescribed drugs with abuse potential are those prescribed for anxiety, pain, and insomnia, including benzodiazepines, and it has been reported that the most commonly abused drugs in elderly patients admitted for treatment were sedative-hypnotics and opioids. Substance abuse problems in this population are often misdiagnosed because of the patients' denials and the providers' own biases and beliefs.

In the older adult population, substance use disorders can be early or late onset. *Early-onset use* is defined as a substance use disorder that occurs before the age of 65 years. This group makes up two-thirds of elderly substance-dependent patients. *Late-onset use* is associated with the development of stressful life situations, including loss of a partner, changes in living situation, retirement, or social isolation. Lily is in the late-onset group and had a clear stressor leading to her substance use disorder.

Unfortunately, there is a general lack of evidence-based treatment approaches for this population. Treatment may depend on the patients' overall medical conditions and stability and functional impairment. The need for detoxification and inpatient rehabilitation with extensive and intensive outpatient therapy should be considered in this group of patients. Psychotherapy, motivational interviewing, and cognitive-behavior therapy have been shown to have positive outcomes for this group of patients.

Because of the risks associated with the use of prescription medications in the elderly population, explicit criteria have been developed to catalogue medications that cause adverse drug events in older adults because of their pharmacological properties and the physiological changes of aging. The American Geriatrics Society recommends not using benzodiazepines and other hypnotics as a first-line treatment for insomnia in this age group. Sedative-hypnotics should be used with care in this population.

Although Lily did not abuse any other substances, in one study individuals who were hospitalized for benzodiazepine-involved reasons were much more likely than those hospitalized for other substances to report the abuse of another substance (95% versus 54.4%; Substance Abuse and Mental Health Services Administration 2011). Older adults, however, were generally more likely to report benzodiazepines as their only substance of abuse: 11.5% of patients age 55 years or older indicated that benzodiazepines were their only substance of abuse, compared with about 3%–5% of those ages 12–44 and 8% of those ages 45–54.

Treatment of sedative, hypnotic, or anxiolytic use disorder can involve pharmacological and behavioral strategies. Lily was able to complete detoxification from sedatives during a 5-day inpatient stay, but this is not always possible for patients who have high levels of physiological dependence. For those patients, longer-term outpatient detoxification strategies should be employed. Patients should be switched from short-acting agents such as alprazolam to longer-acting agents such as clonazepam, with the dose then gradually decreased over a period of several weeks to even months. Physicians should monitor patients for symptoms of withdrawal and provide patients with education about more serious withdrawal symptoms that would necessitate a hospital visit.

Although there are effective evidence-based medications for the treatment of sedative withdrawal, there are no medications approved by the U.S. Food and Drug Administration for the chronic treatment of sedative, hypnotic, or anxiolytic use disorder. The success seen with replacement or agonist therapy for the treatment of opioid and tobacco use disorders has not been replicated in sedative, hypnotic, or anxiolytic use disorder. It is unclear why agonist therapy does not work in these individuals.

After the initial stabilization period, patients should engage in ongoing outpatient substance abuse treatment, as is done with other drugs of abuse, in order to develop recovery skills. Psychotherapy remains the mainstay of treatment for sedative disorders, with evidence supporting the use of cognitive-behavior therapy, relapse prevention therapy, and 12-step facilitation techniques.

For individuals with co-occurring anxiety or sleep disorders that may have been a contributing factor to their substance abuse, ongoing treatment of these conditions is essential to successful substance abuse treatment. When pharmacological treatment is used, agents with low abuse liability, such as SSRIs, buspirone, and gabapentin, should be employed for treatment of anxiety. For insomnia, sedating antidepressants, antihistamines, and melatonin agonists have markedly decreased risk for abuse.

Psychosocial interventions for co-occurring disorders are an important part of the recovery process as well. Patients should engage in psychotherapy for these disorders and learn about the relationship of psychiatric symptoms to substance use. Given the high occurrence of sleep disturbances in patients with a history of sedative use disorders, education about sleep hygiene should be provided as well.

Lily's case suggests multiple areas for prevention and treatment of sedative use disorders. Given the relatively high potential for abuse and frequent comorbid substance use, patients should be screened for alcohol and other substance use disorders. Prescribing physicians should ensure that patients dispose of leftover medication properly and monitor prescriptions closely so they are aware when patients are seeking early refills or visiting multiple providers. Screening and planning for mental health and medical issues early in the treatment process can help ensure that these issues can be effectively addressed and may in some cases eliminate or reduce the need for sedative medications.

Key Points

- Use of sedative-hypnotics as first-line agents for insomnia in the elderly population should be avoided.
- When sedative-hypnotics are used for the treatment of insomnia, patients should be carefully assessed for risk factors for misuse of the medication or dependence. This assessment should continue during the treatment process.
- The nonbenzodiazepine medications have not been definitively demonstrated to be without risk, and there is little data about their long-term effects.
- Treatment of co-occurring mental illness is essential to successful substance abuse treatment.

References

American Geriatric Society: American Geriatrics Society updated Beers criteria for potentially inappropriate medication use in older adults. J Am Geriatr Soc 60:616–631, 2012

American Society of Addiction Medicine: Principles of Addiction Medicine, 2nd Edition, Text Revision. Chevy Chase, MD, American Society of Addiction Medicine, 1999

Bogunovic O: Substance abuse in aging and elderly adults. Psychiatric Times 9:1–6, 2012

McCall W: Sleep in the elderly: burden, diagnosis, and treatment. J Clin Psychiatry 6:9–17, 2004

Substance Abuse and Mental Health Services Administration: Detailed Tables: National Estimates, Drug-Related Emergency Department Visits for 2004–2009. Rockville, MD, Office of Applied Studies, 2010. Available at: http://www.samhsa.gov/data/2k13/DAWN2k10ED/DAWN2k10ED.htm. Accessed October 27, 2013.

Substance Abuse and Mental Health Services Administration: The TEDS Report: Substance Abuse Treatment Admission for Abuse of Benzodiazepines. Rockville, MD, Substance Abuse and Mental Health Services Administration, June 2011

Questions

8.1 Which of the following can be a potentially life threatening symptom associated with sedative, hypnotic, or anxiolytic withdrawal?

A. Myocardial infarction.
B. Stroke.
C. Seizure.
D. Respiratory depression.

The correct answer is C.

Respiratory depression can be associated with sedative, hypnotic, or anxiolytic intoxication but not withdrawal.

8.2 Which of the following substances of abuse has been successfully treated using agonist therapy as a chronic treatment?

A. Cannabis.
B. Heroin.
C. Cocaine.
D. Crystal methamphetamine.
E. Diazepam.

The correct answer is B.

Agonist, or replacement, therapy has been successfully used as a chronic treatment of opioid use disorder and nicotine use disorder. This works by providing a substance similar to the drug of abuse in order to prevent cravings and drug use. This strategy has not been demonstrated to be successful for other substances, including sedatives. The reasons for this remain unclear. Agonist therapy is used for detoxification from sedatives.

8.3 Which of the following is *not* useful in the treatment of individuals with sedative, hypnotic, or anxiolytic use disorder?

A. Sleep hygiene for patients with insomnia.
B. Cognitive-behavior therapy for substance use disorders.
C. Cognitive-behavior therapy for co-occurring psychiatric disorders.
D. Naltrexone to relieve cravings for sedatives.
E. Long-acting benzodiazepines for management of withdrawal.

The correct answer is D.

Naltrexone has been used for cravings for alcohol and opioids but has not been proven to be effective for sedatives.

8.4 Which of the following risk factors is not associated with development of substance abuse in older adults?

A. Male gender.
B. Social isolation.
C. History of substance abuse.
D. History of mental illness.
E. Exposure to prescription drugs.

The correct answer is A.

Older females are at greater risk of developing drug abuse.

8.5 Which of the following is false regarding benzodiazepine receptor agonists?

A. They exert their effect at the GABA receptor.
B. They include classical benzodiazepines as well as nonbenzodiazepines.
C. They are available only by prescription.
D. They have a relatively uniform duration of action of about 8 hours.
E. They are among the most prescribed medications.

The correct answer is D.

These medications vary widely in their duration of action and elimination half-lives from a few hours to several days.

CHAPTER 9

Stimulants

Sex, Drugs, and Techno: Gay Men and Crystal Methamphetamine

Joe Ruggiero, Ph.D.

UNDERSTANDING the context and meaning of a client's drug or alcohol use can be crucial when treating a person who uses substances. Often, drug treatment focuses on the cessation of drug use without truly understanding the role of the substance in the client's life. The meaning of a person's use includes such factors as the individual's motivations, internal experience and expectations of the drug, the setting in which he or she uses, and how social an experience it is (Denning 2000). Each person has a unique relationship to his or her drug(s). In this chapter I describe the treatment of a client with stimulant use disorder and emphasize how important it is to consider his motivations, the context of his use, and what drew him to the substance. Only through understanding this can we help clients make changes in their substance use as well as help them improve their quality of life.

In the early 2000s, researchers started documenting the rise in methamphetamine ("crystal") use in New York City among gay and bisexual men (Halkitis 2009). Originally, this substance was prevalent in the western United

States, primarily with women. However, during the early 2000s it became more prevalent on the East Coast among gay and bisexual men. Methamphetamine, like cocaine, inhibits the reuptake of dopamine, but it also increases dopamine and serotonin release. With methamphetamine, users experience a high that is much more powerful and longer lasting than that of cocaine. In addition, the aftermath, or the "crash," lasts longer, and users are more at risk for greater depression, suicidal ideation and acts, and psychosis when compared with cocaine users (Levounis and Ruggiero 2006).

Reback (2005) interviewed gay men to understand why they are drawn to methamphetamine. She found that gay men use methamphetamine in order to better their sexual experiences, decrease anxiety about HIV, and make themselves more comfortable with sex. HIV-positive gay men who are using methamphetamine and going online find that they do not need to discuss their status because it is often stated in computer profiles or because it is assumed that they are positive. This helps them avoid the possible anxiety related to speaking about these issues and negotiating sex practices as well as possibly facing rejection. In addition, methamphetamine may help gay men deal with the shame and internalized homophobia of having sex with other men.

Because crystal works for a prolonged period of time, users often want to have sex for hours and will have multiple partners, which places them at greater risk for HIV. Even if they start by having safer sex, it is difficult to continue to do so with a large number of partners. In addition to the intense sexual experience, gay men also feel a tremendous interpersonal connection to other men when using. This can be especially powerful considering the alienation many gay men experience. Often, when authors discuss gay men and crystal, they focus so much on sex that they ignore the connection and "intimacy" gay men may be attempting to experience when using. Some clients who use crystal talk about the desire to connect as well as the desire for sex.

In order to work with gay men who use crystal, it is imperative to make the treatment culturally sensitive and to address issues of identity, coming out, HIV, sex, and sexuality. The client treated in the following case example was working in treatment specifically designed for gay men using methamphetamine (see Figure 9–1), with the hope that it would allow him to more easily discuss those issues.

Clinical Case

Peter is a 36-year-old white gay male who came to treatment for methamphetamine use disorder after his family performed an intervention regarding his use. Unfortunately, he experienced the intervention as very shaming and felt coerced to consider treatment options. The intervention involved bringing him and his family together with a clinician and confronting him on his methamphetamine use. He had had no idea the intervention was going to occur and was wary of

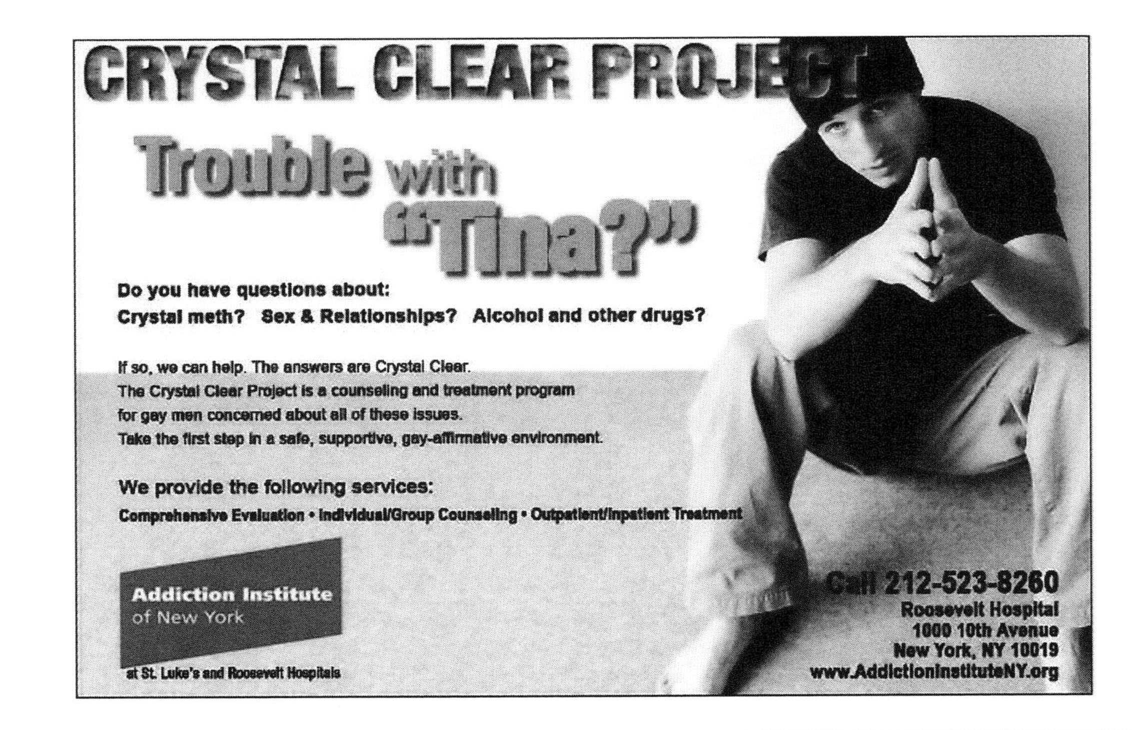

FIGURE 9–1. An example of a program that specifically addresses gay men using methamphetamine.
Source. Courtesy of the Addiction Institute of New York.

treatment, but he realized he had some kind of problem and opened up during the consultation.

Peter was born and raised in upstate New York in a fairly conservative town. As an adolescent, he realized he was gay and had great social struggles in school although he was clearly quite intelligent and performed well academically. He grew up and worked in a family business that required a great deal of physical labor. He felt quite inept at work and was often chastised by his three older brothers and ignored by his father. In high school, he was "outed" by other adolescents because he was having a relationship with a male schoolmate. Being outed caused a great deal of shame for him regarding his sexual orientation because it was so public and made his family and peers aware of his being gay. He said that his relationship with an older sister changed dramatically after he came out. She was his one ally, and he felt a distance that continued to the present day. Peter's mother had separated from his father when he was 7 years old, and he had had little contact with her; as he progressed in therapy, he realized this was probably because of an alcohol problem she had had.

Peter left his town to go to college and did quite well, eventually earning an MBA. He worked in banking in New York City and struggled with being in a very conservative work environment where he felt many were biased against him because of his sexual orientation. He also believed that his orientation was limiting his options to advance in his firm, and he thus grew increasingly dissatisfied with work.

During this time, Peter developed a pattern of coming home from work after a stressful day and going on the Internet, cruising the chat rooms and Web sites to find partners for anonymous sex. He felt that his "sexual compulsivity" (as he called it) predated his drug problem. He would often go on the Internet for hours and eventually started frequenting sex clubs as well. Peter felt alone and alienated at work and in the city, and he struggled to connect socially. Online, he found a community that embraced him.

As his sexual behaviors continued, Peter was exposed to methamphetamine. He did not have a great awareness of the drug and started using it without knowing what he was doing. At that time, around the year 2000, there was little information in the media about methamphetamine, even though it was quite prevalent on the West Coast. It was common at that time for gay men who presented with methamphetamine addiction to state that they did not know what they were using but that they had been exposed to it when they were having sex. Peter began by smoking methamphetamine but eventually used it through injection. He found that sex felt more powerful when he was high. He also experienced incredible connections between himself and other men while under the influence. This had a significant effect on Peter considering how alienated he had often felt in New York City and with other men. He now felt connected to a social world that was linked by drug use and sexual behavior.

Peter preferred to anally penetrate men when having sex, and crystal allowed him to feel quite powerful when doing so. Again, this was compelling because he had felt so insignificant during his life in his other relationships with men. Methamphetamine makes men feel sexual but hinders getting an erection; thus, during his sexual experiences, Peter would have receptive anal sex at times, putting himself at risk for HIV. When went to the consultation, he was concerned that he might be HIV positive but thought that he could not handle the news if he were.

Postexposure prophylaxis was not yet available, so there were no medical interventions that could be used to avoid seroconversion. Peter told himself that he would be able to stop his use of methamphetamine, and he tried to stop but was unable to achieve more than 2 weeks of sobriety. As his use progressed, he felt more distance between himself and his friends. He canceled and missed social gatherings with friends. His use had started as weekend binges but had escalated, and he began to miss days at work. His employers thought he needed to move on, partially because of behaviors related to his drug use. He confided about his drug use to a cousin, who then told his family members, and they staged the intervention.

Discussion

Substance Use Diagnosis

Methamphetamine, like other stimulants, does not involve the physiological withdrawal often associated with other substances such as alcohol, benzodiazepines, and opioids. Many clients continue to use crystal because they want to avoid the depressive crash associated with withdrawal, which can also include insomnia or hypersomnia, hyperphagia, vivid unpleasant dreams, and psychomotor retardation or agitation. In cases of severe insomnia or agitation, a short course of benzodiazepines can be used. In addition to psychological withdrawal, other diagnostic criteria associated with a stimulant use disorder (see Box 9–1) are also present in Peter's case, such as ongoing use despite knowledge of adverse consequences (e.g., work problems, family strain, possible seroconversion, and loss of friendships). Men who use crystal will begin to spend hours online searching for men with whom to have sex and use drugs. Eventually, weekend partying will extend into the week. Their weekends will consist of using, going online, and having sex, thus meeting the criteria for preoccupation and excessive time spent using or around using. For many people who use substances, there can be a ritual connected to the use from which it is hard to disengage, in addition to the time spent actively using. In Peter's case his use progressed from smoking to intravenous use and also from weekend to weekday use. He also had less time for social engagements and was less available at work (criteria of important social, occupational, and recreational activities given up or reduced). Peter alienated friends, who distanced themselves from him. He felt he could stop on his own and made attempts to stop but was unsuccessful.

Box 9–1. DSM-5 Criteria for Stimulant Use Disorder

A. A pattern of amphetamine-type substance, cocaine, or other stimulant use leading to clinically significant impairment or distress, as manifested by at least two of the following, occurring within a 12-month period:

1. The stimulant is often taken in larger amounts or over a longer period than was intended.
2. There is a persistent desire or unsuccessful efforts to cut down or control stimulant use.
3. A great deal of time is spent in activities necessary to obtain the stimulant, use the stimulant, or recover from its effects.
4. Craving, or a strong desire or urge to use the stimulant.
5. Recurrent stimulant use resulting in a failure to fulfill major role obligations at work, school, or home.
6. Continued stimulant use despite having persistent or recurrent social or interpersonal problems caused or exacerbated by the effects of the stimulant.
7. Important social, occupational, or recreational activities are given up or reduced because of stimulant use.
8. Recurrent stimulant use in situations in which it is physically hazardous.
9. Stimulant use is continued despite knowledge of having a persistent or recurrent physical or psychological problem that is likely to have been caused or exacerbated by the stimulant.
10. Tolerance, as defined by either of the following:
    a. A need for markedly increased amounts of the stimulant to achieve intoxication or desired effect.
    b. A markedly diminished effect with continued use of the same amount of the stimulant.

    Note: This criterion is not considered to be met for those taking stimulant medications solely under appropriate medical supervision, such as medications for attention-deficit/hyperactivity disorder or narcolepsy.
11. Withdrawal, as manifested by either of the following:
    a. The characteristic withdrawal syndrome for the stimulant (refer to Criteria A and B of the criteria set for stimulant withdrawal, DSM-5 p. 569).
    b. The stimulant (or a closely related substance) is taken to relieve or avoid withdrawal symptoms.

    Note: This criterion is not considered to be met for those taking stimulant medications solely under appropriate medical supervision, such as medications for attention-deficit/hyperactivity disorder or narcolepsy.

Specify if:

In early remission: After full criteria for stimulant use disorder were previously met, none of the criteria for stimulant use disorder have been met for at least 3 months but for less than 12 months (with the exception that Criterion A4, "Craving, or a strong desire or urge to use the stimulant," may be met).

In sustained remission: After full criteria for stimulant use disorder were previously met, none of the criteria for stimulant use disorder have been met at any time during a period of 12 months or longer (with the exception that Criterion A4, "Craving, or a strong desire or urge to use the stimulant," may be met).

Specify if:

In a controlled environment: This additional specifier is used if the individual is in an environment where access to stimulants is restricted.

Coding based on current severity: Note for ICD-10-CM codes: If an amphetamine intoxication, amphetamine withdrawal, or another amphetamine-induced mental disorder is also present, do not use the codes below for amphetamine use disorder. Instead, the comorbid amphetamine use disorder is indicated in the 4th character of the amphetamine-induced disorder code (see the coding note for amphetamine intoxication, amphetamine withdrawal, or a specific amphetamine-induced mental disorder). For example, if there is comorbid amphetamine-type or other stimulant-induced depressive disorder and amphetamine-type or other stimulant use disorder, only the amphetamine-type or other stimulant-induced depressive disorder code is given, with the 4th character indicating whether the comorbid amphetamine-type or other stimulant use disorder is mild, moderate, or severe: F15.14 for mild amphetamine-type or other stimulant use disorder with amphetamine-type or other stimulant-induced depressive disorder or F15.24 for a moderate or severe amphetamine-type or other stimulant use disorder with amphetamine-type or other stimulant-induced depressive disorder. Similarly, if there is comorbid cocaine-induced depressive disorder and cocaine use disorder, only the cocaine-induced depressive disorder code is given, with the 4th character indicating whether the comorbid cocaine use disorder is mild, moderate, or severe: F14.14 for mild cocaine use disorder with cocaine-induced depressive disorder or F14.24 for a moderate or severe cocaine use disorder with cocaine-induced depressive disorder.

Specify current severity:

Mild: Presence of 2–3 symptoms.

305.70 (F15.10) Amphetamine-type substance
305.60 (F14.10) Cocaine
305.70 (F15.10) Other or unspecified stimulant

Moderate: Presence of 4–5 symptoms.

304.40 (F15.20) Amphetamine-type substance
304.20 (F14.20) Cocaine
304.40 (F15.20) Other or unspecified stimulant

Severe: Presence of 6 or more symptoms.

304.40 (F15.20) Amphetamine-type substance
304.20 (F14.20) Cocaine
304.40 (F15.20) Other or unspecified stimulant

Source. Reprinted from the *Diagnostic and Statistical Manual of Mental Disorders,* 5th Edition, Washington, DC, American Psychiatric Association, 2013. Used with permission. Copyright © 2013 American Psychiatric Association.

Other Psychiatric Diagnoses

In addition to diagnosing stimulant use disorder, (most likely) severe, other psychiatric diagnoses often need to be addressed when working with men using methamphetamine. At times, methamphetamine users may become quite psychotic and paranoid. Some crystal users may hold on to the delusions that are present even as they start to get sober, which can be challenging when a clinician tries to engage them in treatment. Many methamphetamine users present themselves at emergency departments while psychotic and may need an antipsychotic early in treatment.

Depression can also result when a person is crashing or withdrawing from crystal. Clients who have depressive and suicidal histories may be at higher risk for a suicide attempt or gesture. Peter had to address his ongoing depression after a period of sobriety. He felt that he was always depressed even before he stopped using and described a low-grade chronic depression consistent with a diagnosis of persistent depressive disorder (dysthymia). After 9 months of sobriety, he felt he did not enjoy things in his life and agreed to a psychopharmacological consult. Some clients who use methamphetamine will feel depressed even after a significant period of sobriety because of the dopamine depletion they experience. It was unclear how much Peter's depressive symptoms were substance induced, but taking an antidepressant was helpful. Although clients have the right to choose whether or not to take medications, it can be difficult to deal with the low energy, anhedonia, and depressive symptoms without medication. Some clients may feel triggered to use in order to deal with this depressive state and may need a great deal of support to keep them from using in order to feel better. Clients may also need psychoeducation because the crash can be so extended and confusing to some.

Peter told the clinician that his "sexual addiction" predated his drug use. The diagnosis of sexual addiction is quite controversial. One school of thought led by Patrick Carnes (2001) likens it to drug addiction in that it involves reaching out for something external to adjust internal mood states and anxiety. However, opponents of this school of thought such as Ley (2012) have discussed the lack of empirical evidence for such a disorder and the morality and judgment that are often entangled in this diagnosis. In DSM-5 (American Psychiatric Association

2013), a decision was made to not include this diagnosis under non-substance-related addictive disorders. Regardless of the diagnostic classification, it is important to address the issues of sexual behaviors in treatment because they are distressing to the client. As the reader can see, addressing sexual issues was crucial in Peter's case.

Cultural Considerations

As we go on to discuss treatment, it is important to acknowledge the cultural context of treatment. A therapist needs to have a certain comfort level for working with gay men when treating this population. Such issues as internalized homophobia, coming out, and gay identity are important to discuss and assess with gay men who use methamphetamine. There can be a great deal of shame connected to drug use and sexual behaviors, and the therapist needs to create as nonjudgmental a space as possible. Clinicians should be clear about their tolerance for hearing about sexual orientation, sex, and drug use. It can be damaging for clients to experience any prejudice, judgment, or intolerance within the treatment space. When treating clients in groups, the therapist needs to be aware of any discriminatory experiences that happen within the space between gay and heterosexual clients. In addition, it is also important to understand how LGBT friendly and inviting one's clinic or office environment is. Even if the therapist is supportive, the client also needs to feel some safety in the clinic or office where the therapy takes place.

Treatments

Unfortunately, besides using an antidepressant for some methamphetamine users, there are no approved chemical interventions to manage cravings or withdrawal for stimulant users. Psychosocial interventions and relapse prevention models are useful. Halikitis (2009) stated that a cognitive-behavior therapy (CBT) such as the Matrix Model (Anglin and Rawson 2000) can be especially helpful. This model involves a CBT protocol that not only addresses relapse prevention skills such as identifying triggers and managing cravings but also includes family education and drug monitoring. The Friends Research Institute (Shoptaw et al. 1998) developed a culturally sensitive version of the Matrix Model for gay men who use methamphetamine. Their manualized protocol includes relapse prevention techniques and also deals with identity issues by discussing life as a sober gay man, life as an HIV-positive gay man, and coming out as a sober gay man. They include gay events and establishments in their manual such as gay pride parades, bars, and bathhouses. One session involves exploring and defining sexual behaviors the client feels comfortable with when using and when sober and the connection of other drugs as they relate to sex. Although some clients have other chemical addictions in addition to crystal, it is not uncommon for others to have never abused a drug before. Therefore, an examination of the role of various substances in one's life can be important. Some men may feel alienated by the assumption that they should be completely sober when they enter treatment, and the pros and cons of this choice should be discussed with them.

Reback et al. (2004) studied 263 gay and bisexual methamphetamine users who were randomly placed into one of four conditions: a CBT group, a contingency management (CM) group, a combination of CBT and CM, and a culturally sensitive protocol. All groups showed reduction in methamphetamine use. Although the groups did not differ with regard to level of methamphetamine reduction, the culturally sensitive group had the fastest reduction in unprotected receptive anal intercourse. Often, studies focus only on abstinence, but clients may show progress in other areas as well. There are ways in which clients progress and their quality of life improves that may not be reflected when focusing only on drug use. This finding is important when considering prevention of HIV and other sexually transmitted diseases.

In his review of psychosocial approaches to methamphetamine use, Halikitis (2009) also discussed the importance of CM, which involves rewarding the user with vouchers for attendance or negative urine toxicology results. This is intended as a way to engage the client, to reinforce not using, and to counter the reinforcing nature of drug use. The vouchers can be used for material items, food, movies, and so on. Studies have found that this intervention can improve retention and result in more negative urine analyses. CM has been shown to be as powerful an intervention as CBT.

Although Peter had been in individual therapy for years, his therapist did not feel skilled in addictions and therefore made the referral. Peter felt coerced to have a consultation by his family's intervention, but he agreed to participate in an intensive program and to do individual therapy. When assessing Peter, it became clear that using a motivational interviewing perspective would be especially helpful because his reason for entering treatment was based largely on external pressures (Miller and Rollnick 2002). Motivational interviewing explores the ambivalence that clients have as they enter treatment and normalizes it, which involves rolling with the resistance. In Peter's case it was important to be clear about his options—for example, addiction treatment (inpatient or outpatient), traditional therapy, self-help, or no treatment—and being able to make a choice was crucial for him. He was aware of his drug problem but was suspicious of the treatment field and his family's agenda for him.

Intensive outpatient programs have been found to be a good choice for methamphetamine addiction. The program that Peter joined has specific groups that look at methamphetamine use and gay men and explores issues of sex, sexuality, and homophobia in a safe context. Some clients find that discussing intimate sexual issues in a mixed group can be inhibiting. Peter's family had insisted on his attending inpatient treatment, but he did not want to do so because he thought he needed to find another job. Instead, he wanted to take a leave of absence from his job to work on his drug use and look for another job while in treatment. He agreed that if this did not help, he would consider inpatient treatment. Often, family and others assume that a person will not improve unless he or she goes inpatient. Inpatient stays may help stabilize a person, but they are not always necessary for everyone who enters treatment. If the person who made Peter's assessment had been at all coercive, it could have resulted in Peter's failing to engage in treatment. In addition, he might have been blamed for "not being ready" to go inpatient.

Peter was able to engage in the intensive program and to start creating relapse prevention skills and building sober time. As he spoke to more men in the program who attended self-help groups, he agreed to try Crystal Methamphetamine Anonymous and grew more involved over time. Often, treatment can provide a bridge to self-help for those who find it helpful by first having them explore issues in a context that is mediated by a professional. Peter seemed to be helped by hearing about self-help from others who did not insist on it, thus allowing him to freely explore his program. He went on to engage in self-help and obtain a sponsor.

Peter struggled with his goal of sobriety. He felt that he was not addicted to alcohol or marijuana, which he used socially, but he explored his options in therapy. Clients have different relationships with different substances, and it is important to acknowledge that clients should make choices from a motivational interviewing perspective. Peter chose to be sober from all substances. He worried that if he drank he might call his dealer and use. Although he did not think that smoking marijuana was risky with regard to crystal, he decided to set complete chemical abstinence as a goal. Because he was engaged in self-help, he believed he would connect better to and be accepted by others in his self-help group who were setting the goal of abstinence.

Group therapy and self-help allowed Peter to look at the way he made connections to gay men and to build a support network. Many of his friends had distanced themselves from him because of his use, so he was in need of a more immediate support network. Some gay men who use crystal struggle to have nonsexual relations with the men in self-help and in the program. The treatment program has a rule against romantic and emotional entanglements while in treatment. However, many men are used to sexualizing other men and can struggle to interact in a different way. In the beginning weeks, Peter did have sex with some of the other self-help members but then made a decision to not do so for 6 months. He wanted to work on creating nonsexual connections. He was worried about these relationships going wrong and leading him to distance himself from certain meetings in order to avoid previous sexual partners. Finally, some of the men in the program were also not stable and could lead to his using. At times, men in group therapy can trigger each other in the way they speak about their drug use and sex.

Group therapy can allow gay men to look at how they interact and learn how to make connections to each other in nonsexual ways. It can be healing because they may support each other without physical contact. They can value themselves for things other than being a sexual object or partner. They may also start to understand the barriers that they create in achieving intimacy.

Initially, Peter made a decision not to be tested for HIV because he thought he would not able to deal with the results if they indicated that he was positive. Once he built a support network and felt more confident with his therapists, he was able to get tested and learned he was negative. He was also able to explore in therapy the ways he put himself at risk when he was sexually active both while he was using and before his use. He defined behaviors that he felt comfortable with sexually versus those that he did not feel as comfortable with and explored the ways that he had put himself at risk. As Peter became more sexually active, we would monitor his behaviors and how comfortable he felt with them.

One of the early critical components of Peter's treatment was to identify how to handle his online behaviors and being sexually active. He decided to take a "break from sex" for 60 days and not have anonymous sex. He felt this would allow him to have a foundation of stability. With many men who use crystal, it is important to discuss sex and ways to manage it and to help them set policies about how they want to handle their sexual behaviors because this is such a powerful trigger for them.

After he reached 60 days, Peter began to speak about how to be sexually active without exposing himself to drugs. We discussed ways to be sexually active and which ways exposed him to the risk of using, how much of a risk this was, and how much he was willing to risk the possibility of using. He also wanted to understand what it meant to feel "horny" or feel that he needed sex. There were times when this felt like a physical need, but often it seemed like a way to distract him from what he was feeling or to manage his anxiety. He was able to be active in safer ways that did not expose him to drugs. Peter also started to discuss what it felt like to have sex in an impulsive way that felt similar to his drug urges because he wanted to feel more in control of his sexual behaviors.

Clients whose use is connected to sex often need to redefine sex for themselves and the ways they use sex (e.g., to connect, to fulfill a need, or to manage anxiety). Even clients whose use is not connected to sex may discuss the struggle of sober sex. Some have never had sex when not under the influence of something, and the experience of sober sex can be terrifying. Also, gay men who use crystal may have intense standards of sex such as the idea that sex involves a great many partners or should go on for days. These standards often need to be reevaluated when they are having sex while sober. They may actually have different desires when sober and may need to relearn what they are doing sexually as a sober person. Last, crystal helps men feel confident and disconnect from the anxiety they may experience when having sex, and clients need to learn to manage these feelings without using.

As Peter progressed in therapy and his sobriety, he was able to explore his struggles with building relationships and understanding whether he could have a more intimate relationship with a man. We discussed his barriers to intimate connection with other men beyond sex. Peter often felt unable to have a relationship with a man because he felt inadequate and had internalized the insecurity that he felt as a child with the men in his life. He struggled when dating because he wanted to please and be liked by the other person but often lost himself as he got to know a man. We worked on creating better boundaries in relationships and asserting himself so that he could get his needs met. This work came after he had built a period of sobriety.

Peter also was able to reconnect with his family. It seemed important to have some initial distance from them so that he could focus on caring for himself and get some distance from the intervention. In addition, by allowing Peter to make choices about his treatment and to define how it might look, he was able to own his treatment and did not feel he was "mandated" to seek help. He was better able to feel internally committed to his sobriety.

Early on in treatment Peter made a decision to not receive any psychiatric medications. He had taken zolpidem but had concerns about his abusing it to help him sleep after his crystal use. He also had been given an antidepressant, but he wanted to stabilize to see how he felt. In addition, he believed he had chronic sleep problems. Medication and discussion of sleep hygiene were helpful.

In summary, holistic therapeutic work with Peter involved stabilization, therapy, psychiatric interventions, and self-help support. The work had to be culturally sensitive because of the deep shame that he felt from using drugs and being very active sexually. It is often quite a challenge for both the therapist and the client to create an environment in which gay men can discuss issues of sex and drugs, topics for which they have often been judged and which they have had to hide.

Key Points

- Whenever dealing with any type of substance, it is important to explore the context and the meaning of the substance.
- When working with gay men who use methamphetamine in sexual situations, it is important to help them explore their sexual behaviors as triggers to their use and to define what sexual behaviors they feel comfortable with as they build sober time.

- CBT and CM are two effective psychosocial modalities used for methamphetamine addiction.
- No pharmacological interventions are available, although methamphetamine users often may need an antidepressant to deal with dopamine depletion as they get sober.
- Treatment needs to be culturally sensitive in order to address the context of use. Such issues as sex, HIV, and drug use should be discussed in a nonjudgmental therapeutic space.

References

American Psychiatric Association: Diagnostic and Statistical Manual of Mental Disorders, 5th Edition. Washington, DC, American Psychiatric Association, 2013

Anglin D, Rawson R: The CSAT methamphetamine treatment project: what are we trying to accomplish? J Psychoactive Drugs 32:209–210, 2000

Carnes P: Out of the Shadows: Understanding Sexual Addiction. St. Paul, MN, Hazelden, 2001

Denning P: Practicing Harm Reduction Psychotherapy. New York, Guilford, 2000

Halkitis PN: Methamphetamine Addiction: Biological Foundations, Psychological Factors, and Social Consequences. Washington, DC, American Psychological Association, 2009

Levounis P, Ruggiero J: Outpatient management of crystal methamphetamine dependence: can it be done? Prim Psychiatry 13:75–80, 2006

Ley D: The Myth of Sexual Addiction. Baltimore, MD, Rowan and Littlefield, 2012

Miller WM, Rollnick S: Motivational Interviewing: Preparing People for Change, 2nd Edition. New York, Guilford, 2002

Reback CJ: The Social Construction of a Gay Drug: Methamphetamine Use Among Gay and Bisexual Men in Los Angeles. Los Angeles, CA, AIDS Coordinator for the City of Los Angeles, 2005

Reback CJ, Larsons S, Shoptaw S: Changes in the meaning of sexual risk behaviors among gay and bisexual male methamphetamine abusers before and after drug treatment. AIDS Behav 8:87–96, 2004

Shoptaw S, Reback CJ, Freese TE, et al: Behavioral Interventions for Methamphetamine Abusing Gay and Bisexual Men: A Treatment Combining Relapse Prevention and HIV Risk-Reduction Interventions. Los Angeles, CA, Friends Research Institute, 1998

Questions

9.1 Which of the following is true about methamphetamine and cocaine?

A. Methamphetamine alone impacts the levels of dopamine in the brain.

B. Both cocaine and methamphetamine stimulate dopamine release, but cocaine also impacts reuptake.
C. Cocaine involves a longer and more intense high.
D. Methamphetamine is similar to cocaine in that they both block dopamine reuptake, but methamphetamine also stimulates dopamine release.

The correct answer is D.

The crash after methamphetamine use can be more intense and harder, and the person may be more at risk for greater depression and suicidal behaviors or thoughts.

9.2 Which of the following statements is true regarding psychosocial interventions?

A. Self-help has been proven to be the most effective intervention when working with methamphetamine users.
B. Contingency management (CM) and cognitive-behavior therapy (CBT) are two effective modalities for methamphetamine users.
C. When working with methamphetamine users, it is important to use proven psychopharmacological interventions first to eliminate cravings.
D. All of the above.

The correct answer is B.

There are no psychopharmacological interventions for methamphetamine, and although self-help may be helpful, CM and CBT have been shown to be effective.

9.3 Motivational interviewing involves

A. Confronting the resistance.
B. Confronting denial.
C. Rolling with resistance.
D. None of the above.

The correct answer is C.

Motivational interviewing involves working with ambivalence and does not involve confrontation or denial.

9.4 Methamphetamine

A. Originated in New York City and has yet to spread west.
B. Was originally more common in the West.
C. Is common only among gay men nationally.

The correct answer is B.

Methamphetamine was more common in the West originally and came to the Northeast later on. In the eastern United States, methamphetamine use is more frequently restricted to gay men, whereas it is more widely used in the western United States.

9.5 The following was found when comparing the Friends Research Institute protocol with CM only, the Matrix Model, and both the Matrix Model and CM in gay male methamphetamine users:

A. The protocol was better than all the other modalities with regard to lowering drug use.
B. The protocol led to increases in use.
C. The protocol was less effective in lowering use.
D. None of the above.

The correct answer is D.

The protocol was equally effective as the other conditions but decreased unprotected anal receptive intercourse as well.

CHAPTER 10

Tobacco

From Social Norm to Modern Day Faux Pas

Robbie Bahl, M.D.
Petros Levounis, M.D., M.A.

TOBACCO use has undergone a spectacular transition in our society over the past 50 years. It was once the most popular sign of self-assurance, encompassing our television commercials, newspapers, and airline promotions. Today it is banned from bars, workplaces, and even public parks. The days of looking cool with a cigarette are becoming obsolete. Smoking a cigarette today has a high likelihood of being perceived as unattractive and unhealthy.

Tobacco use disorder is the most common form of chemical dependence in the United States (Box 10–1). Quitting smoking can be difficult and typically requires multiple attempts. There is significant clinical evidence that clinicians can help their patients achieve a smoke-free lifestyle using tactics that range from simple eye contact and conversation to prescription medications.

Smoking cessation brings an abundance of health benefits, even for the long-term, older smoker. In the United States, there has been significant progress toward smoking cessation at the population level. As of 2002, the number of former smokers exceeded the number of current smokers. The problem, however, is far from over. According to the Centers for Disease Control and Prevention and the U.S. Department of Health and Human Services,

Box 10–1. DSM-5 Criteria for Tobacco Use Disorder

A. A problematic pattern of tobacco use leading to clinically significant impairment or distress, as manifested by at least two of the following, occurring within a 12-month period:

1. Tobacco is often taken in larger amounts or over a longer period than was intended.
2. There is a persistent desire or unsuccessful efforts to cut down or control tobacco use.
3. A great deal of time is spent in activities necessary to obtain or use tobacco.
4. Craving, or a strong desire or urge to use tobacco.
5. Recurrent tobacco use resulting in a failure to fulfill major role obligations at work, school, or home (e.g., interference with work).
6. Continued tobacco use despite having persistent or recurrent social or interpersonal problems caused or exacerbated by the effects of tobacco (e.g., arguments with others about tobacco use).
7. Important social, occupational, or recreational activities are given up or reduced because of tobacco use.
8. Recurrent tobacco use in situations in which it is physically hazardous (e.g., smoking in bed).
9. Tobacco use is continued despite knowledge of having a persistent or recurrent physical or psychological problem that is likely to have been caused or exacerbated by tobacco.
10. Tolerance, as defined by either of the following:
    a. A need for markedly increased amounts of tobacco to achieve the desired effect.
    b. A markedly diminished effect with continued use of the same amount of tobacco.
11. Withdrawal, as manifested by either of the following:
    a. The characteristic withdrawal syndrome for tobacco (refer to Criteria A and B of the criteria set for tobacco withdrawal).
    b. Tobacco (or a closely related substance, such as nicotine) is taken to relieve or avoid withdrawal symptoms.

Specify if:

In early remission: After full criteria for tobacco use disorder were previously met, none of the criteria for tobacco use disorder have been met for at least 3 months but for less than 12 months (with the exception that Criterion A4, "Craving, or a strong desire or urge to use tobacco," may be met).

In sustained remission: After full criteria for tobacco use disorder were previously met, none of the criteria for tobacco use disorder have been met at any time during a period of 12 months or longer (with the exception that Criterion A4, "Craving, or a strong desire or urge to use tobacco," may be met).

Specify if:

On maintenance therapy: The individual is taking a long-term maintenance medication, such as nicotine replacement medication, and no criteria for tobacco use disorder have been met for that class of medication (except tolerance to, or withdrawal from, the nicotine replacement medication).

In a controlled environment: This additional specifier is used if the individual is in an environment where access to tobacco is restricted.

Coding based on current severity: Note for ICD-10-CM codes: If a tobacco withdrawal or tobacco-induced sleep disorder is also present, do not use the codes below for tobacco use disorder. Instead, the comorbid tobacco use disorder is indicated in the 4th character of the tobacco-induced disorder code (see the coding note for tobacco withdrawal or tobacco-induced sleep disorder). For example, if there is comorbid tobacco-induced sleep disorder and tobacco use disorder, only the tobacco-induced sleep disorder code is given, with the 4th character indicating whether the comorbid tobacco use disorder is moderate or severe: F17.208 for moderate or severe tobacco use disorder with tobacco-induced sleep disorder. It is not permissible to code a comorbid mild tobacco use disorder with a tobacco-induced sleep disorder.

Specify current severity:

305.1 (Z72.0) Mild: Presence of 2–3 symptoms.
305.1 (F17.200) Moderate: Presence of 4–5 symptoms.
305.1 (F17.200) Severe: Presence of 6 or more symptoms.

Source. Reprinted from the *Diagnostic and Statistical Manual of Mental Disorders,* 5th Edition, Washington, DC, American Psychiatric Association, 2013. Used with permission. Copyright © 2013 American Psychiatric Association.

- Approximately 43.8 million people in the United States, or 19.0% of all people age 18 years or older, smoke cigarettes: 21.6% of men and 16.5% of women (Centers for Disease Control [CDC] 2012).
- Cigarette smoking is the leading cause of preventable death (CDC 2002). One of every five deaths is caused by smoking (CDC 2008; U.S. Department of Health and Human Services 2004, 2010).

Addressing smoking cessation is not something the clinician looks forward to. It is a difficult subject because today everyone knows that smoking is "very bad for you." Smokers, especially long-term smokers, are aware of the negative consequence of smoking, are likely to have tried quitting a few times on their own, and perhaps now have given up on the thought of quitting. For some people, smoking is a way of life. They wake up and immediately smoke. They met their spouse while smoking. They spend breaks at work socially smoking and discussing the day's events. Stopping such a routine poses an obvious health benefit, but it comes at a significant cost: it is a major sacrifice to most patients' lifestyles and social norms.

Achieving smoking cessation can take multiple visits, conversations, medications, and lifestyle and environment changes. Reaching a patient's goal on the first try is unlikely. Patients relapse on average eight times before true tobacco cessation is reached. Relapse commonly happens because of stress, weight gain, or withdrawal symptoms (Box 10–2). Examples of withdrawal symptoms include irritability, anxiety, difficulty concentrating, and increased appetite.

In this chapter, we outline the best evidence-based methods for tobacco cessation, allowing patients to reap the benefits of a smoke-free life.

Clinical Case

Leo, a 67-year-old man, came to the office with the chief complaint of chronic cough and exercise-induced shortness of breath. He said that the cough occurs three times a week while he is sleeping. It wakes him up at night two or three times a week. Changing positions in bed or sleeping in a chair does not improve his symptoms. He denied any edema symptoms. In addition, Leo stated that the cough happens when he exerts himself. His cough gets much worse when he decides to use the steps at work. He has been using the elevator to go up even one floor for the past 6 months. His cough is nonproductive and does not induce vomiting. Sometimes he can hear a whistling noise from his lungs when he is having these breathing difficulties. The only relief he gets at work is when he uses two puffs of his wife's albuterol inhaler. At home, he used his grandson's nebulizer for albuterol treatments about 10 times in the past 6 months.

Leo has a past medical history of hypertension, hyperlipidemia, peripheral vascular disease, pneumonia, and osteoarthritis. His pneumonia resulted in a two-night hospital stay 2 years ago. He had a left total knee replacement surgery 4 years ago. Leo's mother and father have passed away; his father died of a sudden myocardial infarction and his mother of trauma secondary to a motor vehicle accident. Both of his parents had been one-pack-per-day smokers throughout their entire lives. Leo does not have any siblings. He lives with his wife of 45 years in a senior development in Wilkes-Barre, Pennsylvania, and works as a courier at a printing plant.

Leo has smoked one pack of cigarettes a day for the past 35 years. He tried to quit four times in the past using different nicotine replacement therapy (NRT) products. Each time, he lasted no more than 2–3 weeks on NRT and then went back to smoking. He has no other history of substance use. His wife also smokes one pack per day. Leo walks at work but does not exercise in any other setting. He has two children, both of whom had had childhood asthma, and currently has one grandchild who is 4 years old and was recently diagnosed with childhood asthma. Leo does not have any allergies to foods or medicines. His current medications include hydrochlorothiazide 25 mg/day, atorvastatin (a statin) 40 mg/day, and two to four over-the-counter ibuprofen caplets weekly for knee pain.

Box 10–2. DSM-5 Criteria for Tobacco Withdrawal **292.0 (F17.203)**

A. Daily use of tobacco for at least several weeks.
B. Abrupt cessation of tobacco use, or reduction in the amount of tobacco used, followed within 24 hours by four (or more) of the following signs or symptoms:
   1. Irritability, frustration, or anger.
   2. Anxiety.
   3. Difficulty concentrating.
   4. Increased appetite.
   5. Restlessness.
   6. Depressed mood.
   7. Insomnia.
C. The signs or symptoms in Criterion B cause clinically significant distress or impairment in social, occupational, or other important areas of functioning.
D. The signs or symptoms are not attributed to another medical condition and are not better explained by another mental disorder, including intoxication or withdrawal from another substance.

Coding note: The ICD-9-CM code is 292.0. The ICD-10-CM code for tobacco withdrawal is F17.203. Note that the ICD-10-CM code indicates the comorbid presence of a moderate or severe tobacco use disorder, reflecting the fact that tobacco withdrawal can only occur in the presence of a moderate or severe tobacco use disorder. It is not permissible to code a comorbid mild tobacco use disorder with tobacco withdrawal.

Source. Reprinted from the *Diagnostic and Statistical Manual of Mental Disorders,* 5th Edition, Washington, DC, American Psychiatric Association, 2013. Used with permission. Copyright © 2013 American Psychiatric Association.

Discussion

Cultural and Generational Considerations

Leo is a typical smoker a physician would see in her or his office. This patient meets several criteria for the DSM-5 diagnosis of tobacco use disorder (Box 10–1; American Psychiatric Association 2013). Smoking 20 cigarettes daily for 35 years while fully aware of the medical risks strongly suggests that Leo has a severe form of the illness. He had already been diagnosed with several chronic medical problems that are all caused or worsened by cigarette smoking. Regardless, he continued smoking even in the face of a possible new diagnosis of chronic obstructive pulmonary disease. His addiction to tobacco is a dominant one, exacerbated by the support of society and his immediate surroundings. In this case, the patient is both chemically dependent on nicotine and behaviorally dependent on the everyday regimen of smoking. His mornings start off with a cigarette and a cup of coffee. His work breaks consist of time spent outside smoking with coworkers. He relaxes with his wife on their front porch multiple times a day smoking cigarettes and talking. After every meal, Leo is not at ease without his postprandial dose of tobacco.

In addition, it appears that smoking cigarettes has been an integral part of Leo's life since a very young age. He grew up in a household in which both parents smoked heavily. He watched his father smoke in the morning at the breakfast table. He sat on the porch and played with his toy cars while his parents smoked cigarettes after dinner. Furthermore, the television shows and advertisements that Leo was exposed to as a young child exemplified smokers as hip and successful pillars of society. To Leo, smoking was just as normal as driving, eating, and walking.

Cigarette smoking may be considered one of the most damaging social norms of all time. For a physician to attempt to undo this essential part of a patient's life is challenging. Leo's generation was raised during a time in which the negative medical effects of tobacco smoking were either completely unknown or significantly underappreciated. Cigarettes had no warning labels, and smoking cigarettes with filters was considered a healthy alternative. These days it is common for a doctor treating people like Leo to be several decades his minor and to have great difficulty imagining tobacco's social acceptance of yesteryear. Therefore, developing a patient-physician trusting relationship with mutual understanding of each other's cultural context has emerged as a fundamental component in smoking cessation. Behavioral interventions and motivational interviewing approaches that allow patients to take charge of their own treatment have been shown to be very effective in enhancing people's internal motivation to change their behavior (Levounis and Arnaout 2010).

Pharmacotherapy

Pharmacological therapies have shown good efficacy for achieving smoking cessation. When used in conjunction with behavioral therapies, these medications can be particularly powerful in helping patients live smoke free. Although pharmaceutical options are also effective as monotherapies, they are not intended to be used without initial counseling and discussion.

NRT is typically the first-line pharmacological treatment option for a patient addicted to nicotine. The nicotine patch has the advantage of well-documented efficacy and provides steady transdermal nicotine levels with multiple dosing options. The patch comes in multiple dosages to accommodate a weaning pattern of treatment. A patient smoking one pack of cigarettes a day (or more) initially receives the 21-mg patch daily and should stop smoking at the time when he or she applies the first 21-mg patch. In patients who fail to respond to the 21-mg patch, a higher dose may be warranted. This high dose is used for 6 weeks, and then the patient transitions to the 14-mg patch for an additional 2 weeks. NRT continues with daily application of the 7-mg patch for a final 2 weeks. For breakthrough cravings, patients should be strongly encouraged to use a second form of NRT such as the lozenge, gum, or inhaler options. Abstinence during the first 2 weeks of patch therapy has been highly predictive of long-term cessation. Patients who concurrently stop nicotine and illegal substances also have higher rates of sobriety.

The nicotine transdermal patch needs to be used for approximately 10 weeks, with weaning dosages as described, in order to be effective. Use of NRT beyond 10 weeks is acceptable if the patient needs it to remain abstinent. However, most patients do not use NRT for the full recommended therapeutic duration. When patients state that they "have tried everything," it is helpful to inquire about the details of the duration of each therapeutic trial. In many cases, patients are not able to complete the full recommended trial of treatment, often resulting in a relapse. Of course, it is unclear if strong cravings (and eventual relapse) are the consequences of the premature discontinuation of NRT or vice versa: strong urges to use fuel disappointment and subsequent discontinuation of the medication. As is often said in the street, "Going to the local drugstore and buying some nicotine patches to show the guys at work does not count."

If NRT alone does not produce favorable results, other medications may be tried. Bupropion sustained release has shown significant efficacy and can be used in conjunction with NRT. Bupropion inhibits neuronal reuptake of norepinephrine and dopamine, resulting in decreased cravings for tobacco. In addition, the same medication can treat depression if needed. The recommended target dose of bupropion sustained release is 150 mg twice a day following 3 days of titration with 150 mg once a day.

Another pharmacological option approved by the U.S. Food and Drug Administration (FDA) for smoking cessation is varenicline. Varenicline acts as a partial agonist of $\alpha_4\beta_2$ nicotinic acetylcholine receptors and therefore should not be used in conjunction with NRT outside a research context. It is recommended that varenicline be used for at least 12 weeks at the dosage of 1 mg twice a day after a week-long titration. If a patient has planned a specific quit date, he or she should start medication 1 week prior to the date. If the patient does not have a quit date, then the physician may ask him or her to stop smoking 8–35 days after starting the medication. The most common side effect of varenicline is nausea, which improves if the patient takes the medication with food.

Varenicline and bupropion carry an FDA black box warning of neuropsychiatric symptoms and suicidality. Physicians should discuss this potential side effect with their patients, screen them for suicidal thoughts before starting either medication, follow up during subsequent visits, and discontinue the medication immediately if such symptoms emerge. Research conducted to date, however, indicates that the risks of psychiatric side effects with varenicline are no greater than with the other smoking cessation medications.

The Clinician's Approach

When the topic of smoking cessation is brought up during a medical visit, tension builds in the room and many practitioners feel as though it is a hopeless pursuit. Recent studies, however, have shown that a physician's verbal recommendation to stop smoking is more efficacious than previously assumed. Although it does take multiple efforts by both the patient and the physician to reach the ultimate goal of cessation, the process should be repeated and documented at every visit. "Saying something" about smoking, especially when it comes from a physician, is a powerful clinical intervention that cannot be overestimated. Effective strategies in primary care settings include the following:

1. Make eye contact and ask if the patient smokes cigarettes. If yes, tell him or her to quit.
2. Inquire further into the patient's particular risks and behaviors.
3. Make it a habit to include a patient's smoking status alongside his or her vital signs. If you use electronic medical records, incorporate smoking status in your vital signs by incorporating it in the software. Simply by placing smoking status alongside vital signs, you send a message to your patient that smoking is as important as blood pressure, temperature, and heart rate. In addition, the patient should initially be asked during the nurse's intake and then again during the doctor's visit.
4. Mention the probable negative cosmetic effects of smoking. Remind the patient that smoking expedites the aging process, particularly on the face. Wrinkles and discoloration on the face occur more frequently in smokers because of the vascular effects of smoking. Yellow skin and fingernails are also common. Point out that the odor and appearance of a smoker do not appeal to many people and could stunt the patient's social life and relationship success.

Sometimes, patients with a primary alcohol or drug problem prefer to focus on smoking cessation after their primary addiction is resolved. Practitioners often agree with this response and postpone smoking cessation efforts. However, greater success rates for both the alcohol or drug addiction and nicotine addiction should be expected if both problems are addressed simultaneously.

Psychotherapy

Motivational interviewing and cognitive-behavior therapy (CBT) can be used successfully by either a physician or a counselor to aid in the patient's smoking cessation efforts. If the patient is motivated for treatment, a target quit day may be established at the time of the initial visit to set goals and to organize treatment times. During subsequent visits, the clinician can help the patient identify smoking triggers and make lists of "people, places, and things" that cue the brain to crave tobacco. Some of the worst cravings are experienced first thing in the morning after night-long abstinence from nicotine and subsequent morning miniwithdrawal. CBT techniques can help patients progressively delay the "first cigarette of the day" more and more, with the goal of eventually quitting altogether. Being able to resist smoking right after waking up in the morning is a good prognostic factor.

Medical Comorbidities

Leo has several diagnoses and risk factors related to tobacco addiction. Hypertension and hyperlipidemia, in combination with smoking, significantly increase the risk of heart disease. Smoking also worsens blood pressure and lipid levels. Leo's peripheral vascular disease is directly caused by his smoking and will worsen exponentially with future chronic use. His bout of pneumonia was likely related to his smoking as well. According to the CDC, all chronic smokers should receive the pneumonia vaccine for prevention purposes. In addition, screening for abdominal aortic aneurysms is recommended in male smokers starting at age 50.

In summary, Leo has multiple medical diagnoses that had resulted from smoking, all of which will worsen with continued usage. His risks of heart disease, stroke, and worsening peripheral vascular disease are very high with continued smoking as well. He is almost guaranteed to have coronary artery disease in his future.

Family Considerations

Leo lives with his wife, who is essentially his smoking partner. Encouraging her to quit smoking with him will increase dramatically his chance of quitting. A significant part of their time together is spent smoking, and without smoking, the couple may become bored and feel lost. Therefore, introducing hobbies and recreational activities would help fill the void of nonsmoking time. Simple walks would be a good place to start.

Discussing the negative effect of Leo's smoking on his grandchild may also help bring the reality of tobacco use disorder as family illness to the forefront. Secondhand smoke is a risk factor for asthma and is likely the cause of his grandchild's respiratory diagnoses. Even the presence of smoke particles on clothing, furniture, and other household items, sometimes referred to as thirdhand smoke, has a negative effect on a child's respiratory function. It seems that everyone in Leo's family has been affected by the addiction.

Key Points

- Talk to your patient about smoking cessation at every patient encounter.
- Start pharmaceutical treatment with NRT, then advance to oral medications.
- Focus on your patient's lifestyle and suggest changes that promote a smoke-free environment.
- Augment pharmacotherapy with behavioral therapy, motivational interviewing, and counseling.
- Address smoking cessation simultaneously with other substance use disorders.
- Conceptualize tobacco use disorder as a family illness.

References

American Psychiatric Association: Diagnostic and Statistical Manual of Mental Disorders, 5th Edition. Washington, DC, American Psychiatric Association, 2013

Centers for Disease Control and Prevention: Annual smoking-attributable mortality, years of potential life lost, and economic costs—United States, 1995–1999. MMWR 51:300–303, 2002

Centers for Disease Control and Prevention: Annual smoking-attributable mortality, years of potential life lost, and productivity losses—United States, 2000–2004. MMWR 57:1226–1228, 2008

Centers for Disease Control and Prevention: Current cigarette smoking among adults—United States, 2011. MMWR 61:889–894, 2012

Levounis P. Arnaout B: Handbook of Motivation and Change: A Practical Guide for Clinicians. Washington, DC, American Psychiatric Publishing, 2010

U.S. Department of Health and Human Services: The Health Consequences of Smoking: A Report of the Surgeon General. Atlanta, GA, U.S. Department of Health and Human Services, Centers for Disease Control and Prevention, National Center for Chronic Disease Prevention and Health Promotion, Office on Smoking and Health, 2004

U.S. Department of Health and Human Services: How Tobacco Smoke Causes Disease: The Biology and Behavioral Basis for Smoking-Attributable Disease. Atlanta, GA, U.S. Department of Health and Human Services, Centers for Disease Control and Prevention, National Center for Chronic Disease Prevention and Health Promotion, Office on Smoking and Health, 2010

Questions

10.1 On average, how many attempts at smoking cessation does it take to successfully quit?

A. 2.
B. 5.
C. 8.
D. 10.

The correct answer is C.

The average number of quit attempts for a chronic smoker before succeeding is eight. This fact is helpful to keep in mind for both patients and clinicians. Relapse is very common, and both parties can benefit from remembering that it may take several attempts before achieving stable sobriety and a smoke-free life.

10.2 For polysubstance users, which addiction should be addressed and treated first?

A. Alcohol.
B. Opioids.
C. Tobacco.
D. Benzodiazepines.
E. All of the above.

The correct answer is E.

Tobacco cessation is best addressed simultaneously with other substance use disorders. It has been shown that higher success rates for cessation of both tobacco and illicit drug use are achieved when both substances are treated at the same time.

10.3 Smoking cessation decreases the risks of which of the following diseases?

A. Heart disease.
B. Chronic obstructive pulmonary disease.
C. Cerebral vascular accident (stroke).
D. Peripheral vascular disease.
E. All of the above.

The correct answer is E.

Smoking cessation hosts many health benefits at any age. People addicted to tobacco are at increased risk of all of the listed medical diagnoses. Although, in general, scare tactics achieve mixed results, a physician telling his or her patients that they are at increased risk for almost every major disease may change their mentality and help facilitate smoking cessation.

10.4 Nicotine replacement therapy (NRT) is contraindicated with which of the following medications?

A. Aspirin.
B. Bupropion.
C. Metoprolol.
D. Varenicline.
E. Lisinopril.

The correct answer is D.

Varenicline and NRT should not be prescribed simultaneously because varenicline, being a partial agonist, blocks $\alpha_4\beta_2$ nicotinic acetylcholine receptors, thus rendering them unavailable for NRT. NRT can be used with any of the other medications listed above when treating a patient for tobacco use disorder.

10.5 At what age should smoking cessation be encouraged in your patients?

A. 18.
B. 21.
C. 50.
D. 65.
E. At all ages.

The correct answer is E.

Smoking cessation should be encouraged at all ages. In terms of reduced morbidity and mortality, adolescents and young adults will reap the greatest benefit from quitting. The elderly will also benefit from smoking cessation because of restoration of lung function and overall improvement of respiratory comfort level. Better sleep and decreased cancer risk may be particularly meaningful to elderly patients.

CHAPTER 11

Other (or Unknown) Substances

The Brave New World of Bath Salts and Other Synthetic Drugs

Petros Levounis, M.D., M.A.
Michael Ascher, M.D.

IN recent years, tales of the negative sequelae associated with a new group of designer drugs known as "bath salts" have been gaining widespread media attention, causing concern for lay people, lawmakers, insurance companies, the U.S. Drug Enforcement Administration, and mental health professionals alike. Until recently, these drugs were available in local head shops and gas stations, but they are now sold online and via drug dealers. Bath salts are often marketed under such brand names as Red Dove, Bliss, Blue Silk, Zoom, Blizzard, Cloud Nine, Ocean Snow, Lunar Wave, Vanilla Sky, Ivory Wave, White Lightning, Scarface, and Hurricane Charlie. Thousands of patients across the country are utilizing emergency medical services for treatment related to the use of these drugs, which are broadly classified under the category of "unknown substances."

"Bath salts" are synthetic variants of cathinone (β-keto phenethylamine, or *khât)*, a naturally occurring compound isolated from the leaves of the *Catha edulis* plant found in East Africa. Cathinone is structurally identical to amphetamine except for a single carbonyl bond at the β carbon. About 10 synthetic cathinone stimulants have been developed, marketed, and distributed across the world. In order to circumvent drug abuse legislation, they have been sold as "bath salts," "herbal incense," "plant food," or "insect repellent" and labeled "not for human consumption" to avoid U.S. Food and Drug Administration (FDA) scrutiny. Although cathinone is a Schedule I substance in the United States, synthetic derivatives with slight modifications continue to be produced by "underground chemists," making the substances difficult to study and regulate. Some of these synthetic cathinone derivates are legal and are found in medicinal compounds such as bupropion, diethylpropion, and pyrovalerone. At the time of this publication, at least 43 states and Puerto Rico have enacted legislation to ban substituted cathinones.

The majority of the unregulated cathinone derivatives that have been marketed in the past few years are ring substituted. Some products are also likely to contain a mixture of different chemicals. Some of the most prevalent cathinone derivatives include mephedrone (4-methyl-methcathinone), methylenedioxymethcathinone (MDMC, methylone), methylenedioxypyrovalerone (MDPV), and α-pyrrolidinopropiophenone (PPP). Depending on the particular substance, the effects are said to be similar to cocaine, amphetamine, or 3,4-methylenedioxymethamphetamine (MDMA, "ecstasy").

Structurally, the newest bath salts such as methylone and MDPV incorporate both the β-keto moiety of the cathinones and the methylenedioxy moiety of ecstasy (see Box 11–1) on the basic amphetamine molecule. See Figures 11–1, 11–2, 11–3, and 11–4 for the chemical structures of cathinone, ecstasy, methylone, and MDPV, respectively.

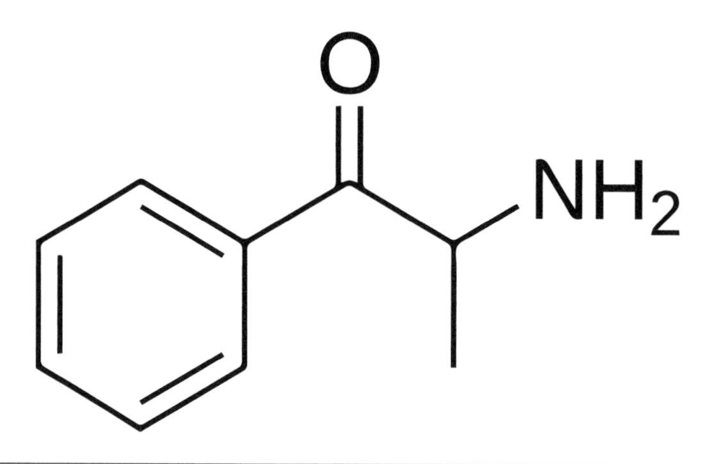

FIGURE 11–1. Chemical structure of cathinone (*khât*).
Source. Wikipedia.

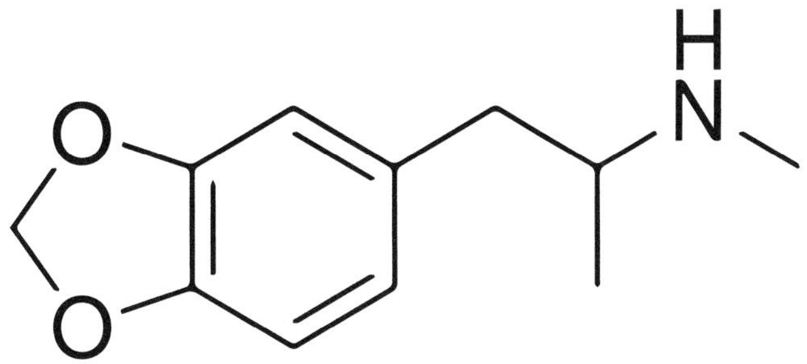

FIGURE 11–2. Chemical structure of methylenedioxymethamphetamine (MDMA, "ecstasy").
Source. Wikipedia.

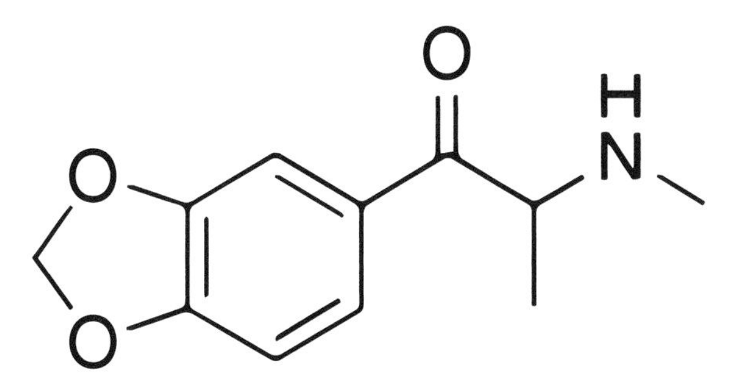

FIGURE 11–3. Chemical structure of methylenedioxymethcathinone (MDMC, methylone).
Source. Wikipedia.

Mephedrone and MDPV are often distributed as white powders packaged in small packets of 500 mg and sell for about $25. Doses of about 25 mg produce the desired effects of improved attention and energy as well as euphoria that last for 2–3 hours in most individuals. Some users compulsively redose to maintain the effects. These drugs are typically administered orally, intranasally, or intravenously. Standard urine toxicology tests do not detect cathinones.

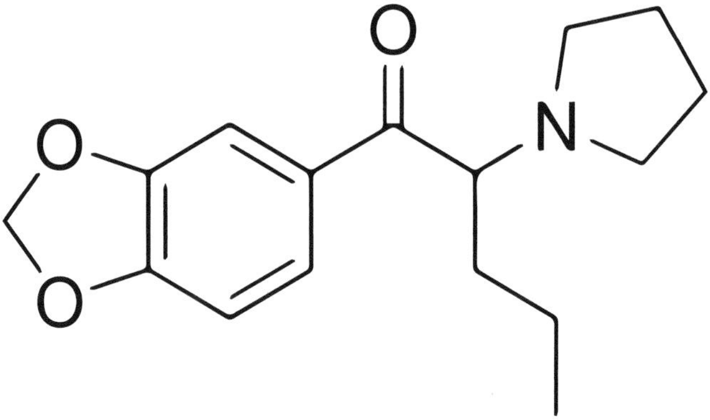

FIGURE 11–4. Chemical structure of methylenedioxypyrovalerone (MD-PV).

Source. Wikipedia.

Box 11–1. DSM-5 Criteria for Other (or Unknown) Substance Use Disorder

A. A problematic pattern of use of an intoxicating substance not able to be classified within the alcohol; caffeine; cannabis; hallucinogen (phencyclidine and others); inhalant; opioid; sedative, hypnotic, or anxiolytic; stimulant; or tobacco categories and leading to clinically significant impairment or distress, as manifested by at least two of the following, occurring within a 12-month period:

1. The substance is often taken in larger amounts or over a longer period than was intended.
2. There is a persistent desire or unsuccessful efforts to cut down or control use of the substance.
3. A great deal of time is spent in activities necessary to obtain the substance, use the substance, or recover from its effects.
4. Craving, or a strong desire or urge to use the substance.
5. Recurrent use of the substance resulting in a failure to fulfill major role obligations at work, school, or home.
6. Continued use of the substance despite having persistent or recurrent social or interpersonal problems caused or exacerbated by the effects of its use.
7. Important social, occupational, or recreational activities are given up or reduced because of use of the substance.
8. Recurrent use of the substance in situations in which it is physically hazardous.

9. Use of the substance is continued despite knowledge of having a persistent or recurrent physical or psychological problem that is likely to have been caused or exacerbated by the substance.
10. Tolerance, as defined by either of the following:
    a. A need for markedly increased amounts of the substance to achieve intoxication or desired effect.
    b. A markedly diminished effect with continued use of the same amount of the substance.
11. Withdrawal, as manifested by either of the following:
    a. The characteristic withdrawal syndrome for other (or unknown) substance (refer to Criteria A and B of the criteria sets for other [or unknown] substance withdrawal, DSM-5 p. 583).
    b. The substance (or a closely related substance) is taken to relieve or avoid withdrawal symptoms.

Specify if:

In early remission: After full criteria for other (or unknown) substance use disorder were previously met, none of the criteria for other (or unknown) substance use disorder have been met for at least 3 months but for less than 12 months (with the exception that Criterion A4, "Craving, or a strong desire or urge to use the substance," may be met).

In sustained remission: After full criteria for other (or unknown) substance use disorder were previously met, none of the criteria for other (or unknown) substance use disorder have been met at any time during a period of 12 months or longer (with the exception that Criterion A4, "Craving, or a strong desire or urge to use the substance," may be met).

Specify if:

In a controlled environment: This additional specifier is used if the individual is in an environment where access to the substance is restricted.

Coding based on current severity: Note for ICD-10-CM codes: If an other (or unknown) substance intoxication, other (or unknown) substance withdrawal, or another other (or unknown) substance–induced mental disorder is present, do not use the codes below for other (or unknown) substance use disorder. Instead, the comorbid other (or unknown) substance use disorder is indicated in the 4th character of the other (or unknown) substance–induced disorder code (see the coding note for other (or unknown) substance intoxication, other (or unknown) substance withdrawal, or specific other (or unknown) substance–induced mental disorder). For example, if there is comorbid other (or unknown) substance–induced depressive disorder and other (or unknown) substance use disorder, only the other (or unknown) substance–induced depressive disorder code is given, with the 4th character indicating whether the comorbid other (or unknown) substance use disorder is mild, moderate, or severe: F19.14 for other (or unknown) substance use disorder with other (or unknown) substance–induced depressive disorder or F19.24 for a moderate or severe other (or unknown) substance use disorder with other (or unknown) substance–induced depressive disorder.

Specify current severity:

305.90 (F19.10) Mild: Presence of 2–3 symptoms.
304.90 (F19.20) Moderate: Presence of 4–5 symptoms.
304.90 (F19.20) Severe: Presence of 6 or more symptoms.

Source. Reprinted from the *Diagnostic and Statistical Manual of Mental Disorders,* 5th Edition, Washington, DC, American Psychiatric Association, 2013. Used with permission. Copyright © 2013 American Psychiatric Association.

The symptoms of bath salt intoxication include significant sympathetic stimulation and altered mental status. Users report feelings of euphoria, increased sex drive, and increased motivation (see Box 11–2). Symptoms can also include agitation, panic attacks, paranoia, hallucinations, hyperthermia, anorexia, muscle spasms, chest pain, hypertension, and tachycardia. Patients can develop life-threatening arrhythmias, cardiac arrest, seizures, stroke, cerebral edema, rhabdomyolysis, and renal failure. Anecdotal evidence suggests that many users become dangers to themselves and others and are at high risk for self-mutilation, suicide attempts, and homicidal activity. Withdrawal symptoms include nasal congestion, fatigue, and insomnia (see Box 11–3). Long-term effects are still unknown because these drugs are relatively new. Some early research indicates that bath salts may have a significant addiction potential, although more studies are needed (Gunderson et al. 2013).

Clinical Case

Benjamin is a 29-year-old white single male who presented to the emergency department with a chief complaint of "Get me out of here!" The patient was disheveled and diaphoretic with significant psychomotor agitation and intense eye contact. He was loud, belligerent, and paranoid and required four-point restraints while lying on a stretcher. He was very difficult to interview and his attention was compromised. The patient was unable to settle down and was not responsive to verbal redirection.

Police reported that they were called after a young woman's neighbor reported hearing "chilling loud screams" and a "scuffle" next door. When police arrived, they broke down the door and found Benjamin and the young woman in a physical struggle. The woman was also being evaluated and treated for cuts and bruises in the medical department.

The resident on call swiftly searched the electronic hospital medical records and learned that the patient was receiving medication management in the outpatient psychiatric department. The chart indicated that Benjamin works as a high school math teacher and had been treated for attention-deficit/hyperactivity disorder (ADHD) and generalized anxiety disorder (GAD) for the past 2 years, for which Benjamin was prescribed atomoxetine 100 mg daily for symptoms related to ADHD and citalopram 20 mg daily for anxiety. He had never been hospitalized for psychiatric reasons, and he did not have any significant medical problems. There was no history of head injuries, seizures, or other neurological conditions. His cognitive baseline status was normal. Benjamin had never experienced any major depressive, manic, or psychotic symptoms in the past. He had never experienced panic attacks or symptoms consistent with agoraphobia, obsessive-compulsive disorder, or posttraumatic stress disorder. He denied any dissociative symptoms. He said he drinks "a few bottles of beer a week" but had no history of delirium tremens, blackouts, seizures, or withdrawal symptoms. He occasionally snorts cocaine "socially" and smokes marijuana "once in a while." His chart did not indicate any other history of substance misuse. Benjamin had never been aggressive toward his sexual partners in the past, and he had no history of violence. He has no current or previous documented legal problems or arrests. He has no reported allergies and no family history of any mental health issues.

The nurses were able to take blood and urine samples from Benjamin after administering an intramuscular injection consisting of haloperidol 5 mg, lorazepam 2 mg, and diphenhydramine 25 mg for significant agitation. His vital signs remained elevated, and he was hypertensive (150/100), with a pulse rate of 117 bpm and a temperature of 99.0°F. His electrocardiogram (EKG) showed sinus tachycardia with QRS 86 ms and QTc 450 ms.

The standard urine and blood toxicology results came back negative for cocaine, amphetamine, marijuana, phencyclidine (PCP), opioids, and benzodiazepines. Alcohol levels were negligible, and Benjamin's blood urea nitrogen (BUN) and creatinine levels were elevated at 26 mg/dL and 2.29 mg/dL, respectively. The rest of his comprehensive metabolic panel and complete blood count were within normal limits. Creatinine phosphokinase (CPK) levels were elevated at 400 U/L. Urinalysis was within normal limits.

The resident learned that the young woman receiving treatment in the medical emergency department was 19 years old, and her name was Kelly. She was very thin with bleached-blond hair, a nose ring, and multiple tattoos. She met Benjamin on an Internet dating site, and they had arranged to meet at a coffee shop in the neighborhood after talking to each other online on only a few occasions. She stated that they went back to her parents' house to "hook up" because her parents were away. On further questioning, the resident discovered that Kelly had purchased a substance called "Cloud Nine" over the Internet and had encouraged Benjamin to try it so he could "relax" because he seemed "real edgy." After they started becoming intimate, he started "to freak out" and began "trying to suffocate [her] with a pillow while scratching, spitting, and biting [her]."

Benjamin's presumptive diagnosis was intoxication with "unknown substance," and urine and blood samples were sent to a commercial laboratory for identification. It was ultimately determined through the use of gas chromatography/mass spectroscopy that Benjamin's blood sample was positive for MDPV. Benjamin was treated supportively and within 72 hours was stable to be discharged to police custody.

Box 11–2. DSM-5 Criteria for Other (or Unknown) Substance Intoxication

A. The development of a reversible substance-specific syndrome attributable to recent ingestion of (or exposure to) a substance that is not listed elsewhere or is unknown.
B. Clinically significant problematic behavioral or psychological changes that are attributable to the effect of the substance on the central nervous system (e.g., impaired motor coordination, psychomotor agitation or retardation, euphoria, anxiety, belligerence, mood lability, cognitive impairment, impaired judgment, social withdrawal) and develop during, or shortly after, use of the substance.
C. The signs or symptoms are not attributable to another medical condition and are not better explained by another mental disorder, including intoxication with another substance.

Coding note: The ICD-9-CM code is **292.89.** The ICD-10-CM code depends on whether there is a comorbid other (or unknown) substance use disorder involving the same substance. If a mild other (or unknown) substance use disorder is comorbid, the ICD-10-CM code is **F19.129,** and if a moderate or severe other (or unknown) substance use disorder is comorbid, the ICD-10-CM code is **F19.229.** If there is no comorbid other (or unknown) substance use disorder involving the same substance, then the ICD-10-CM code is **F19.929.**

Source. Reprinted from the *Diagnostic and Statistical Manual of Mental Disorders,* 5th Edition, Washington, DC, American Psychiatric Association, 2013. Used with permission. Copyright © 2013 American Psychiatric Association.

Discussion

Diagnosis

Substance misuse is a frequent cause of patients presenting with severe agitation in the emergency department. With increased access to information over the Internet, people can now easily obtain different synthetic substances for recreational use.

In the case presented in this chapter, Benjamin was a 29-year-old male brought to the emergency department by police with psychotic and violent agitation. His vitals were elevated, and his EKG showed sinus tachycardia, suggesting a sympathetic response. His CPK and BUN/creatinine were elevated, suggesting muscle breakdown and kidney dysfunction, respectively. All of his other laboratory results, including standard urine drug screening, failed to suggest any substance intoxication, infection, or encephalopathy. Ultimately, outreach to collateral sources (Kelly) and a good history were the keys to developing the preliminary diagnosis of "bath salts" intoxication (Penders 2012; Penders and Gestring 2011). The diagnosis was confirmed only a few days later when blood tests came back positive for MDPV after undergoing gas chromatography/mass spectroscopy testing. Unfortunately, the emergency department did not have access to rapid enzyme-linked immunosorbent assay testing that could have confirmed the diagnosis earlier (Lehner and Baumann 2013).

The clinical picture is similar to that of crystal methamphetamine, PCP, and MDMA delirium or intoxication. Less likely diagnoses to consider include brief psychotic disorder, dementia, delirium due to another medical condition, and substance withdrawal.

In DSM-5 (American Psychiatric Association 2013), the cathinones (including *khât* plant agents and synthetic chemical derivatives) are classified under other (or unknown) substances, despite the fact that these drugs produce primarily stimulant effects. This classification points to the complex properties of the cathinones as part strong stimulants, part hallucinogens, and part PCP-like substances.

Box 11–3. DSM-5 Criteria for Other (or Unknown) Substance Withdrawal **292.0 (F19.239)**

A. Cessation of (or reduction in) use of a substance that has been heavy and prolonged.
B. The development of a substance-specific syndrome shortly after the cessation of (or reduction in) substance use.
C. The substance-specific syndrome causes clinically significant distress or impairment in social, occupational, or other important areas of functioning.
D. The symptoms are not attributable to another medical condition and are not better explained by another mental disorder, including withdrawal from another substance.
E. The substance involved cannot be classified under any of the other substance categories (alcohol; caffeine; cannabis; opioids; sedatives, hypnotics, or anxiolytics; stimulants; or tobacco) or is unknown.

Coding note: The ICD-9-CM code is 292.0. The ICD-10-CM code for other (or unknown) substance withdrawal is F19.239. Note that the ICD-10-CM code indicates the comorbid presence of a moderate or severe other (or unknown) substance use disorder. It is not permissible to code a comorbid mild other (or unknown) substance use disorder with other (or unknown) substance withdrawal.

Source. Reprinted from the *Diagnostic and Statistical Manual of Mental Disorders,* 5th Edition, Washington, DC, American Psychiatric Association, 2013. Used with permission. Copyright © 2013 American Psychiatric Association.

Treatment

Treatment of acute bath salt intoxication is primarily supportive and focuses on counteracting the sympathetic overstimulation. Patients are treated with intravenous benzodiazepines, intravenous fluids, and in some cases, restraints to prevent harm to self and others. Patients are placed on fall and seizure precautions as well as constant one-to-one observation. Clinicians sometimes also consider using low-dose antipsychotics for prominent perceptual disturbances and dangerous behavior.

The clinical presentation can often be complicated when the patient has coingested other substances, most notably crystal methamphetamine or other stimulants (Levounis 2014). As always, reaching out to potential collateral sources (including friends of the patient, acquaintances, loved ones, and the primary care clinician) and taking a careful history typically turn out to be well-rewarded efforts. Bath salts are not detected by the standard urine toxicology screenings, and overdoses can be potentially life threatening if not treated promptly.

Although there is very little published research specifically addressing the treatment of cathinone or other designer drug use disorders (Gunderson et al. 2013), extensive experience in the psychosocial treatments of substance use disorders can be quite informative. There is good reason to believe that a number of interventions shown to be helpful in the treatment of alcohol, sedative, stimulant, and opioid use disorders can also be applied to the treatment of these new drugs of abuse. In addition to traditional individual and group drug counseling, there are established behavioral treatments, including cognitive-behavior therapy, relapse prevention therapy, the community reinforcement approach, multidimensional family therapy, motivational interviewing, and motivational contingency management (Levounis and Arnaout 2010). Partial hospitalization, intensive outpatient programs, and a wide range of inpatient rehabilitation programs are available for people with substance use disorders. An option for patients with more severe problems is a residential treatment program, such as therapeutic communities, which can be very effective. Many patients will find it helpful to immerse themselves in 12-step programs. There are also groups for those who have both medical issues and substance dependence as well as specialized programs that cater to gay, lesbian, bisexual, and transgender patients; senior citizens; women; and dual diagnosis patients (Levounis and Ruggiero 2006).

Pharmacological treatments, on the other hand, have to be tailored to the specific drug of abuse. Because the only FDA-approved pharmacological treatments (available as of the time of writing of this book) are for alcohol, nicotine, and opioid use disorders, little can be gained by looking to medications for the treatment of problems associated with these new designer drugs. However, a practitioner would be greatly helped by knowing the closest "prototype" drug behind each of these new agents, especially when evaluating treatment options for medical emergencies. For example, some of the most common pairs are

- Bath salts (prototype: methamphetamine)
- Spice/K2 (prototype: cannabis)
- Krokodil (prototype: morphine)
- Ketamine (prototype: phencyclidine)
- Gamma-hydroxybutyric acid (GHB) (prototype: γ-aminobutyric acid) (Lee and Levounis 2008)

In the absence of specific research on a drug, the practitioner can make an educated guess in the management of acute intoxication and withdrawal syndromes by consulting the existing evidence that applies to the "prototype" drug.

Key Points

- Bath salts are a group of designer drugs that are synthetic derivatives of β-keto phenethylamine (cathinone).
- Bath salt users report feelings of euphoria, increased sex drive, and increased motivation.
- Patients with cathinone intoxication typically present with sympathomimetic symptoms, which can lead to a medical emergency with significant agitation, psychosis, hyperthermia, muscle spasms, hypertension, and tachycardia.
- Cathinone use disorders are classified in DSM-5 under other (or unknown) substance use disorders because of their unique and complex properties as part stimulants, part hallucinogens, and part phencyclidine-like substances.
- Treatment of acute cathinone intoxication is supportive and similar to treatment for cocaine intoxication.
- Although no studies of long-term treatment of bath salt use disorder have been conducted, it is reasonable to recommend motivational interviewing and other psychosocial interventions that have shown evidence of efficacy and safety for the more common substance use disorders.

References

American Psychiatric Association: Diagnostic and Statistical Manual of Mental Disorders, 5th Edition. Washington, DC, American Psychiatric Association, 2013

Gunderson EW, Kirkpatrick MG, Willing LM, et al: Substituted cathinone products: a new trend in "bath salts" and other designer stimulant drug use. J Addict Med 7:153–162, 2013

Lee SJ, Levounis P: Gamma hydroxybutyrate: an ethnographic study of recreational use and abuse. J Psychoactive Drugs 40:245–253, 2008

Lehner KR, Baumann MH: Psychoactive "bath salts": compounds, mechanisms and toxicities. Neuropharmacology 38:243–244, 2013

Levounis P: Case 16.3: addiction, in DSM-5 Clinical Cases. Edited by Barnhill JD. Washington, DC, American Psychiatric Publishing, 2014, pp 257–259

Levounis P, Ruggiero JS: Outpatient management of crystal methamphetamine dependence among gay and bisexual men: how can it be done? Prim Psychiatry 13:75–80, 2006

Levounis P, Arnaout B: Handbook of Motivation and Change: A Practical Guide for Clinicians. Washington, DC, American Psychiatric Publishing, 2010

Penders T: How to recognize a patient who is high on bath salts. J Fam Pract 61:210–212, 2012

Penders T, Gestring R: Hallucinatory delirium following the use of methylenedioxypyrovalerone (MDPV): "bath salts." Gen Hosp Psychiatry 33:525–526, 2011

Questions

11.1 Bath salts contain which chemical?

A. Ketamine.
B. Synthetic cathinone.
C. Lysergic acid diethylamide (LSD).
D. Phencyclidine.

The correct answer is B.

Cathinone is a naturally occurring substance found in the leaves of the *Catha edulis* plant. Synthetic cathinones are derivatives of this compound and are the principal chemicals in bath salts. Bath salts are not known to contain ketamine, LSD, or phencyclidine.

11.2 Which of the following molecules is *not* a cathinone derivative?

A. Methylenedioxymethamphetamine (MDMA, "ecstasy").
B. Methylenedioxypyrovalerone (MDPV).
C. Methylenedioxymethcathinone (methylone).
D. 4-methyl-methcathinone (mephedrone).

The correct answer is A.

MDMA does not contain the β-keto group, which is obligatory in order to be a cathinone derivative and thus a bath salt. Mephedrone, the original bath salt, as well as methylone and MDPV, are all cathinone derivatives.

11.3 Which of the following symptoms is typical of bath salt intoxication?

A. Bradycardia.
B. Respiratory depression.
C. Creatinine phosphokinase elevation.
D. All of the above.

The correct answer is C.

Bath salts act primarily as sympathomimetic agents and thus result in tachycardia, hypertension, and creatinine phosphokinase elevation.

11.4 All of the following treatments are reasonable choices for someone with severe cathinone use disorder *except*

A. Contingency management.
B. Motivational interviewing.
C. Alcoholics Anonymous (AA) facilitation.
D. Office-based buprenorphine.

The correct answer is D.

Contingency management and motivational interviewing have been shown to be safe and effective in the treatment of stimulant use disorders (for both cocaine and crystal methamphetamine problems) and thus are reasonable choices for the treatment of someone addicted to bath salts. AA is, obviously, geared primarily toward patients with alcoholism, but AA's fellowship has also been extremely helpful to many people who struggle with drug addiction. Given its simple message, big structure, worldwide ubiquity, and long history of helping people stay sober, AA may be recommended for any type of addiction. On the other hand, buprenorphine treatment is reserved strictly for patients with opioid use disorder, moderate or severe.

PART III

Non-Substance-Related Disorder

CHAPTER 12

Gambling

The Woman Who Became Tired of Trying to Predict the Future

Mayumi Okuda, M.D.
Silvia Bernardi, M.D.
Carlos Blanco, M.D., Ph.D.

GAMBLING activities are a feature of almost every culture. Although most individuals who gamble do not develop gambling-related problems, 1%–3% of the adult population and even higher proportions of adolescents develop a gambling disorder. According to DSM-5 (American Psychiatric Association 2013), gambling disorder is characterized by a progressive and maladaptive pattern of gambling behavior that leads to loss of significant relationships, job, and educational or career opportunities (Box 12–1). Disordered gambling is associated with substantial individual suffering and societal burden. Few individuals with a gambling disorder seek treatment, and although about half appear to recover on their own at some point in their lives, the rates of relapse are unknown. Although Gamblers Anonymous (GA) is the most popular intervention for individuals with gambling disorder, less than 10% of attendees become actively involved in the fellowship, and overall abstinence rates are low. Several medications have shown promise in the treatment of gambling disorder, but to date, results of randomized trials have yielded mixed results and there are no medications approved by the U.S. Food and Drug Administration (FDA) for this disorder. At present, cognitive-behavior therapy (CBT) has the strongest empirical evidence for the treatment of disordered gambling.

Box 12–1. DSM-5 Criteria for Gambling Disorder **312.31 (F63.0)**

A. Persistent and recurrent problematic gambling behavior leading to clinically significant impairment or distress, as indicated by the individual exhibiting four (or more) of the following in a 12-month period:

1. Needs to gamble with increasing amounts of money in order to achieve the desired excitement.
2. Is restless or irritable when attempting to cut down or stop gambling.
3. Has made repeated unsuccessful efforts to control, cut back, or stop gambling.
4. Is often preoccupied with gambling (e.g., having persistent thoughts of reliving past gambling experiences, handicapping or planning the next venture, thinking of ways to get money with which to gamble).
5. Often gambles when feeling distressed (e.g., helpless, guilty, anxious, depressed).
6. After losing money gambling, often returns another day to get even ("chasing" one's losses).
7. Lies to conceal the extent of involvement with gambling.
8. Has jeopardized or lost a significant relationship, job, or educational or career opportunity because of gambling.
9. Relies on others to provide money to relieve desperate financial situations caused by gambling.

B. The gambling behavior is not better explained by a manic episode.

Specify if:

Episodic: Meeting diagnostic criteria at more than one time point, with symptoms subsiding between periods of gambling disorder for at least several months.

Persistent: Experiencing continuous symptoms, to meet diagnostic criteria for multiple years.

Specify if:

In early remission: After full criteria for gambling disorder were previously met, none of the criteria for gambling disorder have been met for at least 3 months but for less than 12 months.

In sustained remission: After full criteria for gambling disorder were previously met, none of the criteria for gambling disorder have been met during a period of 12 months or longer.

Specify current severity:

Mild: 4–5 criteria met.
Moderate: 6–7 criteria met.
Severe: 8–9 criteria met.

Source. Reprinted from the *Diagnostic and Statistical Manual of Mental Disorders,* 5th Edition, Washington, DC, American Psychiatric Association, 2013. Used with permission. Copyright © 2013 American Psychiatric Association.

Clinical Case

Amanda is a 62-year-old Haitian woman who immigrated to the United States in her 20s. She is married and has two adult children and three grandchildren. At the time of presentation, Amanda had been working as a secretary and was close to retirement. She presented for treatment at a clinic for gambling disorders after having attended a few sessions at GA. At the time of presentation she did not have any prior psychiatric history and did not meet criteria for any other Axis I or Axis II disorders. She did not use alcohol or drugs. She had diabetes but no other general medical illnesses. She was dressed in colorful casual clothes, was cooperative and pleasant, and upon examination her cognition was intact.

Amanda started gambling in Haiti at an early age, occasionally betting small amounts of money on domino games and local lotteries. At that time, her gambling behavior did not have any immediate adverse consequences; however, paralleling the consequences of early onset of substance use in the general population, it may have predisposed her for a gambling disorder in adulthood. At the age of 30, several years after her arrival in the United States, Amanda began to gamble periodically in hopes of improving her financial situation. She began playing slot machines at casinos and gradually began losing increasing amounts of money. By age 40, Amanda would often spend the entire weekend sitting at the slot machines without sleeping and eating only snacks. Amanda would occasionally forget to administer her insulin injections when she was consumed by her activities at casinos. She was able to stop going to casinos when her frequent trips became a source of marital conflict, but a few years later she began to buy lottery tickets, which were available all over the city.

Amanda spent increasing amounts of money buying lottery tickets ever more frequently. She became increasingly preoccupied with thoughts about gambling and with number combinations. She reported having very vivid dreams that she interpreted as depicting number combinations she should play in the lottery. Growing up in Haiti, she had learned to look for symbols in her dreams because in her culture, dreams were believed to convey important life messages often represented by numbers.

Although she was aware that she was losing more money than she was winning, she would often gamble the day after losing money in hopes of winning back ("chasing") her losses. She concealed the extent of her gambling and her financial situation from her family. Her efforts to reduce or stop gambling resulted in irritability and anxiety. Occasionally, she had suicidal ideation but never made any suicide attempts.

As a result of her gambling, Amanda began to experience financial problems. One of her primary motivations for seeking treatment was the constant arguments with her husband about the monetary constraints caused by her gambling activities. She also felt ashamed and guilty about the money she had spent gambling over the years, which constituted most of her retirement savings. Although she had experienced financial difficulties due to the gambling, Amanda neither committed any illegal acts nor relied on others to bail her out of her financial difficulties. Gambling did not interfere with her work and household chores because it took her only a few minutes during the day to purchase tickets at convenience stores located close to her workplace and home. She experienced some mild difficulties concentrating at work during the minutes prior to the lottery deadline, but she never missed days at work and always performed her work well. She did, however, note the impact of the gambling on her social activities. She became socially withdrawn, spending less time with her children and grandchildren. Her irritability had become a source of increasing arguments with her family members.

Irrational beliefs are often at the root of problem behaviors, and identifying them, pointing out their consequences, and progressively challenging them are key aspects of CBT (Okuda et al. 2009). Irrational beliefs in such things as special dates, playing numbers encountered during the day, and lucky days create in some patients a sense of possessing a special knowledge that they believe increases their chances of winning. Those beliefs can be powerful triggers to gambling even after long periods of abstinence and often trigger a relapse.

Amanda began CBT treatment at the clinic for gambling disorders. As part of her treatment, she was encouraged to describe her gambling activities, focusing on the times she experienced urges to gamble. Describing her gambling activities, she talked about the anxiety she experienced before buying lottery tickets and the frustration, shame, and guilt she felt once the results were published and she was confronted by the amount of money she had lost. She was able to track and see how, despite a few wins, the overall result always had been monetary loss and greater debt. She gradually started to feel less excited about thoughts of winning.

Amanda was able to explore with her therapist the intense frustration she experienced on one particular occasion when she had a dream about the winning number but did not feel the dream strongly enough. She hedged her bets rather than put all her money on the winning number. This experience filled her with doubt about her abilities. She started to experience what she believed was her ability to foresee the future in visions and dreams as an unpleasant responsibility. In the past, stressful familial events had also appeared in her dreams before they happened, but she had been unable to influence those events, which was a very painful experience. She realized now that, similarly, "knowing" the correct number did not lead her to win. As a result, her gambling activities were making her financial situation worse.

After learning to identify her triggers for gambling, Amanda began practicing assertiveness and gambling refusal skills. She stopped carrying her list of numbers and avoided conversations about the lottery, which raised her self-esteem and self-efficacy. After achieving some weeks of abstinence, she felt stronger and more confident. Her urges were mild. She was encouraged to spend more time in alternative pleasant activities, such as physical exercise, going out with friends or to church, helping organize holiday festivities, and participating in other community activities. She also spent more time with her husband, children, and grandchildren. Although Amanda had initially reported that her gambling had never affected her work, she noticed that after weeks of abstinence she was completing tasks at work more efficiently. Her abstinence helped improve her relationship with her husband, with whom she now argued less. She was also excited about being able to buy more things for her home and presents for her grandchildren as a result of not spending money on gambling.

Discussion

Diagnosis

The diagnosis of gambling disorder is clear in this case. Amanda started to gamble with increasing amounts of money in order to achieve the desired excitement, and she became irritable when she tried to cut down. Even though she stopped going to casinos, she started buying lottery tickets and continued to be preoccupied with gambling. Her activities also resulted in guilt, anxiety, and occasionally in suicidal ideation. She continued to gamble after losing money in order to chase her losses. She also concealed the extent of her gambling and jeopardized her relationship with her family. She thus met six out of nine DSM-5 criteria for gambling disorder (only four are needed).

The distress and impairment caused by Amanda's gambling behavior is clinically significant. Amanda jeopardized her relationship with her family and lost most of her retirement savings. The new DSM-5 classification modified the name from *pathological gambling* to *gambling disorder* to reduce the stigma associated with the term *pathological.* Note that the new definition also reduced the threshold for the diagnosis from five to four criteria. The criterion of committing illegal acts such as forgery, fraud, theft, or embezzlement to finance gambling has been eliminated in DSM-5. A recent study using data from samples including individuals varying across the spectrum of severity of gambling problems showed that eliminating the illegal acts criterion did not impact internal consistency of the diagnostic criteria and modestly improved variance accounted for by their factor structure (Petry et al. 2013).

Criterion B states that the gambling behavior should not be better accounted for by a manic episode. In cases in which excessive gambling is a symptom of a manic episode, patients will tend to exhibit other symptoms consistent with a manic episode, such as increased energy, diminished need for sleep, and grandiosity. However, disordered gambling can be triggered by mood changes, and thus it may be challenging to distinguish between gambling behaviors in the context of a manic episode and a gambling disorder triggered by mood symptoms. The assessment of the temporal relationship between these symptoms and the gambling behavior might help clarify the appropriate diagnosis.

Individuals with gambling disorder often have psychiatric comorbidity, particularly lifetime comorbidity. Almost three-quarters (73.2%) of individuals with DSM-IV (American Psychiatric Association 1994) pathological gambling have a lifetime comorbid alcohol use disorder, 38.1% have a drug use disorder, 60.4% have nicotine dependence, 49.6% have a mood disorder, 41.3% have an anxiety disorder, and 60.8% have a personality disorder (Petry et al. 2005). Furthermore, associations between alcohol dependence, drug use disorders, nicotine dependence, major depressive episode, and generalized anxiety disorder and DSM-IV pathological gambling seem to be stronger among women than men. In this particular case, except for some anxiety symptoms and irritability, Amanda did not meet criteria for a prior or current comorbid psychiatric disorder, including a manic or hypomanic episode.

Treatment

Different treatment approaches to treat gambling disorders have been studied (Blanco and Bernardi, 2014). Some of these include GA, marital and family treatments, pharmacotherapy, and manual-guided therapies.

Gamblers Anonymous

GA is the most popular intervention for gambling disorders, with some evidence suggesting that it may have beneficial effects in a minority of participants. Studies have indicated high dropout rates (70%–90%), with only 8% of attendees achieving 1 year or more of abstinence. Combining professional therapy and GA may improve retention and abstinence compared with group participation alone, with some studies showing 64% of patients achieving abstinence.

Marital and Family Treatments

Significant others' involvement in treatment for gamblers has been extensively described. GA has a component for significant others, known as Gam-Anon. A study found that GA members whose significant others participated in Gam-Anon did not have higher rates of abstinence. Despite these data, some patients find the involvement of significant others to be useful.

Pharmacotherapy

Several groups of medications, including antidepressants, opioid antagonists, mood stabilizers, and glutamatergic medications, have been examined for the treatment of gambling disorder. Open trials have been promising for several medications, but placebo-controlled trials have yielded more mixed results (Blanco and Bernardi, 2014). At present, there are no FDA-approved medications for the treatment of gambling disorder. Although specific medications may be useful for particular patients, there is an urgent need to advance in our knowledge about the neurobiology of disordered gambling to allow for a more theoretically based development of pharmacotherapy.

Manual-Guided Therapies

Irrational beliefs are often at the root of problem behaviors, and identifying them, pointing out their consequences, and progressively challenging them are key aspects of CBT. CBT manuals generally comprise components of psychoeducation, increasing awareness about cognitive errors, challenging the validity of irrational cognitions, functional analysis, and cognitive restructuring. CBT is intended to help stop gambling behaviors by helping the patient acquire specific skills, facilitating lifestyle changes, and restructuring the patient's environment to increase the reinforcement from nongambling behaviors. Currently, CBT is the treatment with the strongest evidence of efficacy for gambling disorder, with several randomized, controlled trials demonstrating its efficacy (Cowlishaw et al. 2012). These approaches have been shown to help reduce gambling severity, financial loss, and gambling frequency and to increase the likelihood of remission.

Brief motivational interviewing may be another useful strategy for treatment of gambling disorders, particularly in individuals who are ambivalent about entering treatment. Motivational interviewing, either as a stand-alone treatment or in combination with CBT and personalized feedback, has been shown to help decrease financial loss and gambling frequency and to increase the likelihood of remission.

Key Points

- DSM-5 now lists gambling disorder within substance-related and addictive disorders.
- Similar to other addictions, gambling disorder is influenced by the excitement and pleasure that the patient obtains from the behavior.
- In DSM-5 the diagnostic threshold for gambling disorder has been lowered to four criteria.
- The new definition has eliminated the criterion of committing illegal acts such as forgery, fraud, theft, or embezzlement to finance gambling.
- Gambling disorder can co-occur with different psychiatric disorders, with the caveat that gambling behaviors are not part of a manic episode.
- Although different treatment modalities for gambling disorder have been studied, at present CBT approaches have the strongest evidence of efficacy.

References

American Psychiatric Association: Diagnostic and Statistical Manual of Mental Disorders, 4th Edition. Washington, DC, American Psychiatric Association, 1994

American Psychiatric Association: Diagnostic and Statistical Manual of Mental Disorders, 5th Edition. Washington, DC, American Psychiatric Association, 2013

Blanco C, Bernardi S: Treatment of gambling disorder, in Gabbard's Treatments of Psychiatric Disorders, 5th Edition. Edited by Gabbard GO. Washington, DC, American Psychiatric Publishing, 2014

Cowlishaw S, Merkouris S, Dowling N, et al: Psychological therapies for pathological and problem gambling. Cochrane Database of Systematic Reviews 2012, Issue 11. Art. No.: CD008937. DOI: 10.1002/14651858.CD008937.pub2

Okuda M, Balán I, Petry NM, et al: Cognitive-behavioral therapy for pathological gambling: cultural considerations. Am J Psychiatry 166:1325–1330, 2009

Petry NM, Stinson FS, Grant BF: Comorbidity of DSM-IV pathological gambling and other psychiatric disorders: results from the National Epidemiologic Survey on Alcohol and Related Conditions. J Clin Psychiatry 66:564–574, 2005

Petry NM, Blanco C, Stinchfield R, et al: An empirical evaluation of proposed changes for gambling diagnosis in the DSM-5. Addiction 108:575–581, 2013

Questions

12.1 Which of the following is *not* a diagnostic criterion for gambling disorder?

A. Gambling often when feeling distressed.
B. Often returning another day to get even after losing money gambling.
C. Lying to conceal the extent of involvement with gambling.
D. Committing illegal acts to finance gambling activities.
E. Jeopardizing or losing a significant relationship, job, or educational or career opportunity because of gambling.

The correct answer is D.

The criterion of commission of illegal acts to finance gambling activities was removed in DSM-5.

12.2 Approximately what percentage of individuals with a gambling disorder has a lifetime comorbid alcohol use disorder?

A. Less than 1%.
B. 5%–10%.
C. 20%–30%.

D. 40%–60%.
E. More than 60%.

The correct answer is E.

According to a large epidemiological sample, 73.2% of individuals with DSM-IV pathological gambling have a lifetime comorbid alcohol use disorder.

12.3 Approximately what percentage of individuals with a gambling disorder attending Gamblers Anonymous (GA) achieves 1 year or more of abstinence?

A. Less than 1%.
B. 5%–10%.
C. 20%–30%.
D. 40%–60%.
E. More than 60%.

The correct answer is B.

Approximately 8% of GA attendees achieve 1 year or more of abstinence.

12.4 Which of the following treatments has the strongest evidence of efficacy in the treatment of gambling disorders?

A. Gamblers Anonymous (GA).
B. Cognitive-behavior therapy (CBT).
C. Supportive psychotherapy.
D. Case management.
E. Dialectical behavioral therapy.

The correct answer is B.

CBT approaches have the strongest evidence of efficacy in the treatment of gambling disorder. GA is the most popular intervention for gambling disorders, but it seems to benefit only a minority of participants. Supportive psychotherapy, case management, and dialectical behavioral therapy are not evidence-based treatments for gambling disorders.

12.5 In order to make an accurate diagnosis of gambling disorder, gambling behaviors should *not* be better accounted for which of the following psychiatric conditions?

A. Alcohol use disorder.
B. Manic episode.
C. Major depressive disorder.
D. Obsessive-compulsive disorder.
E. Cannabis use disorder.

The correct answer is B.

To make an accurate diagnosis of gambling disorder, excessive gambling should not occur in the context of a manic episode. Alcohol use disorder, major depressive disorder, obsessive-compulsive disorder, and cannabis use disorder can co-occur with a gambling disorder.

PART IV

Condition for Further Study

CHAPTER 13

Internet

Why Are Drug Addicts and People Who Use the Internet Both Called "Users?"

Steven Joseph Lee, M.D.

THE Internet is a ubiquitous tool that has evolved over time and with increasingly complex technologies so that it has become a routine and necessary part of daily life. However, our constant exposure to it, the myriad benefits that it provides us, the immediate gratification it makes possible, and its rewarding pattern of intermittent variable reinforcement are all factors that increase the risk of users developing a pattern of addictive usage. Despite the ongoing controversy as to whether Internet addiction should be considered a clinical entity of its own, many individuals have presented with classic signs and symptoms of a behavioral addiction. The case that follows illustrates the severity of disability that Internet addiction can cause, as well as the complexity of treating this condition.

Clinical Case

David is a 35-year-old white man referred by his longtime psychotherapist for evaluation of anxiety and lifelong difficulties with concentration. He recalled being an intense worrier, even during early childhood, and while coming to terms with being gay during his adolescence, he began feeling depressed and lonely. During high school David had few friends and spent most of his time at home studying. He had great difficulty listening attentively to his teachers during class, and reading assignments were extremely difficult. He spent much of his junior high and high school years sequestered in his room studying because of both his lack of a social life and his need to compensate for his learning difficulties. Through diligent studying, David achieved good grades and was able to go to a well-known East Coast liberal arts college. During college, David came out and met several gay friends. However, he continued to be an anxious worrier, and lectures and homework in college were much harder than in high school, increasing his anxiety. Despite his small group of gay friends, David remained generally socially isolated. He had a family history of several first-degree relatives with major depression and generalized anxiety disorder.

David had been diagnosed with attention-deficit/hyperactivity disorder (ADHD) in kindergarten. However, he was never treated with medication. Instead, he attended special classes, and in high school, the long hours of homework distracted him from lonely evenings and weekends, which he spent by himself in his bedroom. Teachers in elementary school and high school were impressed by David's intelligence, but he never performed up to their expectations for stellar performance. Their comments deepened David's already low self-esteem, and his low self-regard and social isolation continued during college, even after coming out to an accepting family and friends. After college David continued his studies at a New York law school, where he enjoyed the material and had much less difficulty with his academic work. During law school, David earned straight As, but rather than apply for a position at a high-profile New York law firm, he preferred a low-intensity position as a lawyer in the legal department of a large New York City government bureau, where he felt he could work anonymously and be lost, like a small cog in a huge government-run machine.

When David presented for his initial psychiatric evaluation, his chief complaints were anxiety and difficulty focusing at work. As a parenthetical remark at the end of his first appointment, he briefly mentioned that he spent a lot of time on the Internet in the evenings, which sometimes made him tired in the morning for work.

David had always been reluctant to take psychiatric medications, although for the past 2 years, his psychotherapist had been encouraging him to try medications to attenuate both his anxiety and his difficulties with concentration that had prevented him from taking advantage of insight gained from his therapy. After the threat of job loss for poor work performance, David finally became willing to try medication. He started escitalopram 10 mg once a day, initially targeting anxiety alone to see how much of his impairment in concentration was due to anxiety or depressed mood. After 2 months, David's anxiety was much reduced. He felt more at ease in his workplace, and he was more easily able to accept compliments from his coworkers and supervisor, which he had usually shrugged off. His sleep improved, and he left work without the typical anxious ruminations that used to plague him and frequently caused insomnia. Despite the significant decrease in his anxiety, David's problems with concentration continued, and his supervisor occasionally reprimanded him for mediocre performance. Despite also hearing occasional praise from his boss, David was particularly vulnerable to criticism and was devastated whenever he was told that his work was unsatisfactory.

A trial of a methylphenidate (Ritalin) targeting ADHD was titrated up to 10 mg twice a day and resulted in a dramatic improvement in concentration and work performance, which both David and his supervisor noted. However, the medication caused severe anorexia, so it was changed to mixed amphetamine salts extended release, gradually titrated up to 20 mg every morning. Although his concentration remained good, David also reported an increase in libido and felt that he had a compulsive desire for sex that was greater than that with methylphenidate and made him uncomfortable. His amphetamine dosage was decreased to 10 mg every morning, and escitalopram was gradually increased to 20 mg/day to decrease both his libido and his compulsions. Again, as David walked out the door of his appointment, he made a quiet comment that he hoped his medications would help him stay off of Internet sex sites.

Changes in the dosages of escitalopram and mixed amphetamine salts successfully lowered David's libido and decreased his compulsive sexual activity. For the first time, he disclosed some of his sexual life, admitting that previously he had been masturbating three or four times per day, but in the past month this had decreased to one or two times per day. His anxiety decreased further, and he worried less about dating.

Initially, David's changes appeared to be a clinical victory. However, as we explored David's previous allusions to the Internet, he admitted that he had been struggling to bring up this topic at his appointments for a long time. Although he felt a growing concern about his Internet use, he had felt too ashamed to speak about it. During college and law school, David had used computers and the Internet solely as tools to accomplish his work assignments: writing e-mails, searching databases for his homework assignments, and using offline programs, such as word processors and spreadsheets, to complete his work. However, over the past 4 years, David increasingly used the Internet after returning home from work as a way to soothe his feelings of loneliness and anxiety and his self-perceptions of failure. He frequented mostly gay dating and chat sites, exploring his newly open sexual orientation with enthusiasm. Soon he realized that the anonymity of the Internet allowed him to take on different personas—identities of idealized people whom he wished to be. Some identities were wealthy, some were athletic and physically attractive, and most of them were confident and masculine, although one identity was a female, whom David used to flirt with heterosexual men. He never met any of these people in person, and he abruptly stopped communication with those who began to pressure him to meet in person. Rather than working directly on developing areas of his personality, aspects of his appearance, or other areas in his life that he wanted to improve, David could instantly remove his perceived personal defects and take on whatever characteristics he idealized and dreamt would make him a socially successful and desirable person. He gained a sense of mastery over himself that he had never felt before. Meanwhile, he ignored the fact that these changes in identity were merely illusory and he had made no real positive changes to his core personality.

Eventually, David stopped visiting the online dating and chat sites and instead began to visit gay pornography sites. He spent several nights per week online, masturbating while watching pornography, forgetting about working on his own negative self-perceptions and focusing more on pure sexual gratification. His online sexual activities increased after starting Ritalin, which did not bother him because the pornography was pleasurable, and the Ritalin increased the intensity of his libido and sexual compulsions enough that he could overcome his embarrassment and self-doubt. He felt liberated to enjoy the pleasures of online sex sites. However, the anorexia from the Ritalin was dramatic, and after losing 15 lbs he requested a change to extended-release mixed amphetamine salts. Increasing his dosage up to 20 mg every morning resulted in good concentration but also more frequent online sessions of longer duration, and David found himself either tired and performing poorly at work or oversleeping and arriving at work late. Lowering the dosage of amphetamine salts to 10 mg every morning and increasing escitalopram to 20 mg/day helped somewhat, but the Internet sex activities continued to cause problems at work, so the amphetamine salts were discontinued and replaced with atomoxetine, titrated up to 60 mg/day.

Complete discontinuation of stimulants and starting atomoxetine helped David to significantly reduce his online masturbation to weekends only, and during the week he spent his evenings watching television and sleeping a full 7 hours per night. His energy and focus during the daytime improved, and the atomoxetine had an added benefit of decreasing anxiety further.

On David's return for a follow-up visit 3 months later, he reported that his Internet use had gradually increased back to his previous levels, even in the absence of stimulant medication. Intellectually, David realized that Internet pornography and Internet sex disrupted his sleep and his work and interfered with his ability to develop a social or romantic life. However, emotionally, he admitted that he had no desire to stop his behavior. He felt secure that he would eventually find a person online or pornographic material that would be satisfying. On the other hand, David had strong doubts about his ability to have a successful face-to-face social interaction, and his anxiety about working on his real-life social and romantic experiences was high. In comparison, going home in the evenings to his computer felt safe.

David reported that at least three times during the work week he slept only a few hours, spending most of the night online pursuing virtual sex or pornography. When he first began exploring these sites, he was able to masturbate and achieve orgasm quickly, but over time, he required several hours of searching. Sometimes it felt that the search itself was as gratifying as reaching his intended goal of finding a cybersexual partner, and the length of time spent on the Internet grew to most of the night. The mounting tension of watching the clock turn later and later felt as if it gave him fuel. There were several occasions when David fell asleep at work, and he was eventually fired. At that point, David was finally able to fully recognize that his online behavior was an addiction. Once David made this admission, we were able to address his behavior using cognitive-behavior therapy (CBT) focused on addictive behaviors while trying to use David's medication to support his sexual recovery work, as well as his anxiety and ADHD. Addiction-focused CBT was coordinated with David's weekly individual therapist, who provided supportive psychotherapy to reinforce his ego strengths and work on improving self-esteem and addressing sexual orientation issues.

Employing CBT was difficult with David because he felt such a strong compulsion to return to his computer each night, with the powerful reinforcements of sexual gratification and experiences that contributed to his self-esteem, despite fully knowing that his interactions were based on a false self that he projected onto his cyber personas. Also, he continued to have deep self-doubt about the possibility of succeeding in the real-life social arena, and he repeatedly found excuses why he had to postpone CBT homework assignments. We developed treatment strategies examining and addressing David's personal issues and his unique way of interacting with the Internet. Strategies included completing a detailed decision-matrix self-inventory that examined the positives and negatives of Internet use as well as the positives and negatives of stopping Internet use outside of the workplace; keeping David's laptop on his dining room table and not on his bed, where he was more comfortable to lie for hours while surfing sex sites and masturbating; masturbating to mental images *before* turning on his computer to decrease his libido; setting time limits on when David must turn off his computer, including having a friend call him at a certain time or setting an alarm clock to ring at 11:00 P.M. to signal time to turn his computer off.

When these strategies failed, we discussed leaving David's laptop and the keyboard to his desktop computer in a locked drawer at work or in the home of a friend. An initial suggestion of 1 month without Internet use at home was overwhelming, so the time period was reduced to 1 week. When this was still too daunting, the suggested time period was reduced to 1 day to demonstrate to David that he could tolerate a single night without the Internet. Two months passed before he felt ready to attempt surrendering his computer for a single night, which he completed successfully. Each week, the period of abstinence was lengthened by one additional night, and each week the process became easier. The first few days of abstinence were uncomfortable, but we prepared David by prearranging activities for those evenings, preferably low-stress activities involving face-to-face interactions with friends, which were mostly positive experiences that reminded David of the important life experiences that he had been losing to his addiction. These experiences increased his motivation to continue his efforts. By the time David completed 1 full week of abstinence from evening Internet, which included the entire work week as well as the weekend, the intensity of the compulsion to use the Internet dramatically decreased. David himself suggested that he leave his laptop and his desktop keyboard at his office for safekeeping for 1 month without any computer at home. He completed all his Internet tasks, such as personal e-mails, banking, and shopping, at the office before and after his workday, which helped him to avoid any Internet sex sites that would have triggered relapses.

After 1 month, David decided to bring the keyboard to his desktop computer home, although he kept his laptop at the office so that he would not be tempted to bring a computer into his bed. The presence of a working computer at home increased David's thoughts about the Internet in the evenings. He had occasional cravings to visit sex sites, but he did not succumb to his cravings, which were low enough that he was able to employ the other CBT strategies that we had discussed. Such strategies included 1) setting an alarm clock to signal when his desktop computer must be turned off and 2) scheduling evening activities with friends in advance so that he had social obligations, accountability to friends, and positive reinforcement from his face-to-face social interactions, which gradually helped to build his confidence in his social abilities.

David remained stable with regard to his Internet compulsions, but he became increasingly bothered by the sedation caused by atomoxetine as well as the decreased libido and ejaculatory delay cause by escitalopram. Rather than a trial of another traditional stimulant, David cross-tapered from atomoxetine to modafinil, which increased his feelings of compulsion to visit Internet sex sites, so this was changed to bupropion extended release 300 mg/day. This regimen was slightly less effective at treating his ADHD symptoms but lowered his cravings to use the Internet. At the age of 36, David embarked on his first significant romantic relationship, which was exciting, although also anxiety provoking, awakening his old insecurities and negative self-images. As a result, his cravings to use Internet sex sites, his old coping mechanism for anxiety and low self-esteem, increased, with a couple incidents of relapsing to Internet sex. Extended-release alprazolam 0.5 mg twice a day helped to alleviate some of his anxiety, and although he continued to have thoughts about escaping his real-world anxieties to the artificial cyber world, he was able to utilize his CBT skills to maintain his online sobriety. As David's new relationship developed, with careful exploration and encouragement from his individual psychotherapist, David's confidence in himself grew. In addition, he learned a new set of coping skills to deal with his anxieties and felt empowered because he felt he was actively addressing his problems rather than escaping to the Internet.

In general, David's Internet use remained significantly lower than previously, although his relationship with the Internet remained the same: one of constant vigilance for signs that his old patterns of Internet use would return. During times of stress and increased anxiety, thoughts and cravings for Internet use, especially Internet sex, would return. In addition, David had a circadian rhythm sleep disorder with a sleep phase shift delay, with a delayed sleep time and a delayed wake time. He noted that on nights when he lay in bed wide awake, insomnia itself was a trigger for Internet use and Internet sex. After a few trials of medications to help with sleep, David settled on a regimen of strict sleep hygiene, melatonin 1 mg at bedtime, and bright light exposure with a 10,000 lux light box for 30 minutes every morning, which was extremely effective.

David remained sober from inappropriate Internet use for more than 1 year on a regimen of escitalopram 20 mg/day, bupropion extended release 300 mg in the morning, and alprazolam extended release 0.5 mg twice a day. He began taking classes at a local college in preparation to apply to medical school; he was still in a relationship with the person he had met more than 1 year prior; and in general he reported feeling that his life was more interesting, satisfying, and fulfilled. When he broke up with his boyfriend, he was upset but not devastated, and surprisingly, he did not resort to the Internet for comfort. He joined a 12-step group for sex addiction to increase his social support and to help keep himself sober from Internet sex. There he met a number of men who also compulsively used the Internet for sexual gratification. Because so much of today's dating is initiated online, David thoroughly explored the risks and benefits of using Internet dating sites in psychotherapy. He decided to carefully use Internet dating sites on his desktop computer at home, adhering to his self-imposed restrictions. After 6 months he began dating someone new.

Unfortunately, David's new insurance plan at his college did not cover escitalopram, which at the time was available only in nongeneric form. At the advice of his insurance company, he requested that he be cross-tapered from escitalopram to citalopram, titrated up to 80 mg/day. Although it is a related compound, citalopram did not have as robust an efficacy as escitalopram, and the compulsions to use the Internet became stronger, resulting in relapses to Internet sex. David was demoralized and so frustrated by his return to compulsive Internet use that he decided to take a break from medications and psychotherapy. After that he was lost to follow-up, and the status of his Internet addiction is currently unknown.

Discussion

Background

Although networks between computers have existed since the birth of the modern-day computer in the 1950s, large-scale development of computer networking did not begin until the 1970s, and a global networking of computers that was officially dubbed the "Internet" was born in the late 1980s (Tanenbaum 1996). Since then, the impact of the easy availability of information and the development of software to harness that information has profoundly affected global society, changing the way that people learn, communicate, socialize, and conduct business. The Internet has firmly established itself as an indispensable part of modern living, and in modern and developed countries, the vast majority of individuals use the Internet on a daily basis to accomplish routine personal, social, and occupational tasks.

As technology rapidly developed, the Internet became accessible in new ways, including laptop computers, a new generation of cell phones called "smart phones," computer tablets such as the iPad, "smart TVs," and video game machines. With all of these different forms through which information could be received and transmitted, the ways in which the Internet has been able to incorporate itself into people's lives has grown exponentially from basic word processing programs and financial and banking applications to Internet-driven functions as basic as alarm clocks and daily organizational tools. In particular, the Internet has changed the way in which people interact, with social media allowing people to exchange information, join groups of people with similar interests, and publicly post personal, social, or political information. The changes to our culture in the United States, as well as many other countries throughout the world, have been so rapid that most people do not even realize the extent to which the Internet has woven itself into so many aspects of our lives. Losing a cell phone today can mean losing the database that houses most of our personal information, the schedules of our daily lives, the connection through which our jobs and social networks communicate with us, the portal through which we view entertainment, and the computer applications that we routinely use for accomplishing life's basic tasks. The Internet can transform and dramatically streamline the things that we can accomplish, and loss of the Internet or Internet devices can be devastating.

A 2006 study by the Pew Research Center showed that 73% of respondents (corresponding to approximately 147 million adults) were current Internet users, an increase from 66% the previous year (Madden 2006). A later study conducted in 2012 showed that 95% of households with an income of $75,000 or greater are Internet users (Jansen 2010).

Prevalence

Problematic use of the Internet was proposed as early as 1995 by Ivan Goldberg, who satirically compared it with the behavioral addiction of pathological gambling (http://web.urz.uni-heidelberg.de/Netzdienste/anleitung/wwwtips/8/addict.html, accessed April 13, 2013). Since then, however, the concept of Internet use as a true behavioral addiction has grown significantly. As the number of Internet users worldwide has increased, so have cases of people experiencing an impulse or compulsion to use the Internet that is so compelling that it causes significant impairment socially, professionally, sexually, and even physically, as some extreme Internet addicts neglect self-care activities such as eating and sleeping. Estimates of Internet addiction vary widely, particularly between different countries, because of differing penetration of Internet usage into the general population as well as the lack of a single commonly used set of criteria defining Internet addiction. Estimates vary widely from 0.3% to 38% (Chakraborty et al. 2010). A review of studies estimating prevalence in the United States and Europe by Weinstein and Lejoyeux (2010) indicated a prevalence rate between 1.8% and 8.2%.

DSM-5 Diagnosis

Considering how ubiquitous the Internet is, it is surprising how little research exists on Internet use and addiction in the medical literature. The existence of a distinct clinical condition of Internet addiction continues to be debated in the United States, and there is controversy about the inclusion of Internet addiction disorder in formal diagnostic systems (Pies 2009).

Internet gaming disorder is identified in Section III of DSM-5 (American Psychiatric Association 2013, pp. 795–798) as a condition warranting more clinical research and experience before it might be considered for inclusion in the main book as a formal disorder. However, Internet addiction is not included in DSM-5 because of lack of data demonstrating that it is an independent clinical entity rather than a manifestation of another psychiatric disorder, such as depression, anxiety, or obsessive-compulsive disorder (OCD). Perhaps in the future, Internet addictive behavior may be considered as 1) a primary diagnosis, 2) a secondary diagnosis of self-medication to other primary psychiatric conditions, or 3) a maladaptive coping strategy.

As of the writing of this book, there is no uniform definition of Internet addiction, so it is difficult to make reasonable estimates of prevalence of the condition or to meaningfully study responses to various treatment modalities. Some of the more popular terms used to describe the phenomenon of addictive use of the Internet include Internet addiction disorder, problematic Internet use

(Davis 2001), computer addiction, Internet dependence (Dowling and Quirk 2009), compulsive Internet use, and problematic Internet use (Caplan 2002).

Characteristics

Because the types of activities performed on the Internet are so varied, Internet addiction has been subcategorized into five major groups: 1) cybersex addiction, including use of online pornography, adult chat rooms, and adult fantasy role-play sites that may interfere with real-life relationships; 2) cyber relationship addiction, including social networking, chat rooms, and text messaging to the extent that online relationships become more important than real-life nonsexual relationships; 3) Net compulsions, including online gaming, gambling, stock trading, and online auctions; 4) information overload, which describes a general compulsion to surf the Internet and search for information in databases; and 5) computer addiction, which is a non-Internet addictive behavior that involves use of offline computer games and programs to the extent that real-life activities and responsibilities are neglected (Saisan et al. 2013).

Despite the lack of a single agreed-on definition of Internet addiction, most descriptions of problematic Internet use include the following criteria (Tao et al. 2010):

1. Frequently using the Internet for periods of time far longer than originally intended
2. Continuing to use the Internet at the expense of home or work duties
3. Sacrificing sleep in order to continue using the Internet
4. Isolation from family, friends, and romantic or sexual interactions, which have been replaced by online activities or "cyber relationships"
5. Feelings of guilt or lying to others about the extent of one's Internet use
6. Elevation of mood or decrease in depressed or anxious mood states when using the Internet
7. Feelings of depression, anxiety, irritability, anger, or insomnia when unable to access the Internet or when there is a perceived threat to one's ability to use the Internet (withdrawal)
8. Gradually increasing time spent on the Internet in order to maintain the positive mood effects of online activities (tolerance)

China, a country whose skyrocketing economy is transforming the culture of the largest country population in the world, has more than 338 million Internet users. Although this is only a fraction of the 1.35 billion people in China, this minority surpasses the total population of the United States, and in absolute terms, such a great number of people with Internet addiction poses a severe social and economic threat to China. China has been concerned about Internet use for more than a decade, but it is difficult to interpret the real meaning behind Chinese news reports because there is also the confounding issue of the Chinese government's view of the Internet as a threat to the political regime because of the government's spiraling loss of control of information to the Chinese public. Concerns about Internet addiction could actually be a tactic to discourage use of the Internet for political rather than social and health reasons. Nonetheless, anecdotal reports of extreme Internet addiction abound, and they are consistent with reports from other countries. For example, a gaming addict in Chengdu died after playing *Legend of Mir 2* nonstop for 20 hours in a Net club. Two youths from Chongqing, exhausted after 2 days of constant online gaming, passed out on railroad tracks and were killed by an oncoming train. A boy in Qingyuan butchered his father after an argument in which the father tried to limit the boy's excessive Internet usage. The Chinese government took swift action and stopped issuing licenses to new Internet cafes and closed down more than 16,000 illegal Internet establishments in 2004. In 2007, the Chinese government required antiaddiction safeguards, such as mandating that Internet cafes limit customers' game time to 3 hours. In 2009, the Chinese government began discussion of including Internet addiction in its medical establishment as a formal clinical disorder (Stewart 2010). That year, Beijing's Military General Hospital created China's first Internet-addiction treatment center, using a combination of psychotherapy, physical training, and medication. Similar "boot camp" style treatment centers began proliferating throughout China to keep up with the need to address the huge numbers of people who developed severe problems associated with Internet use (Stewart 2010). Despite the possibility that Chinese politics distort estimates of the prevalence and the severity of negative consequences, both South Korea and Taiwan, which do not share China's political agenda, have also declared Internet addiction a major public health threat. In addition, several Asian countries besides China have established Internet addiction treatment centers, including South Korea, Thailand, and Vietnam.

Etiology

There are many theories about the etiology of Internet addiction, such as the cognitive-behavior model of problematic Internet use (Davis 2001); the anonymity, convenience, and escape (ACE) model (Young 1999); the access, affordability, anonymity (Triple-A) engine (Cooper et al. 1999); a phases model of pathological Internet use (Grohol 2011); and a comprehensive model of the development and maintenance of Internet addiction by Winkler et al. 2011), which considers sociocultural factors, biological vulnerabilities, psychological predispositions, and specific attributes of the Internet to explain excessive engagement in Internet activities.

From a behavioral perspective, the Internet engages the user in an interactive pattern that powerfully reinforces learning and repetition in a manner termed *random intermittent reinforcement.* Even more effective than a constant and consistent reward every time a person uses the Internet, the unpredictable pattern of reward is the strongest type of reinforcement to encourage learning and instill a compelling drive to repeat the learned behavior.

Most significantly, the classic pathophysiological theory of addiction, involving dopamine release in the nucleus accumbens and the establishment of aberrant reward pathways, has been demonstrated with Internet use (Bai et al. 2001; Ko et al. 2009).

Assessment

Because there is no official definition of what signs and symptoms are necessary to identify problematic Internet use, many clinical assessment scales have been developed (Demetrovics et al. 2008; Meerkerk et al. 2009; Widyanto et al. 2001; Young 2011; Young and Nabuco de Abreu 2011). To date, the most widely used assessment scale is the Internet Addiction Test (IAT), a 20-item self-administered examination that employs a five-item Likert scale (Young 1998). The IAT screens for Internet addiction and estimates the severity of problematic Internet use. It has been validated in English, French (Khazaal et al. 2008), and Italian (Ferraro et al. 2007) and has been translated into several other languages. The IAT has been employed widely in numerous countries facing the growing problem of Internet addiction.

Treatment

Even without the recognition as a formal clinical entity, enough individuals present with problematic consequences from Internet use that several treatment centers specializing in the treatment of Internet addiction have been established, including the Center for Internet Addiction Recovery, founded by Dr. Kimberly Young, and reSTART (http://www.netaddictionrecovery.com/), a residential treatment program in Seattle, Washington. Other institutions, such as McLean Hospital, a Harvard Medical School affiliate, and the Illinois Institute for Addiction, have developed intensive outpatient treatment programs for Internet addiction recovery. Traditional residential addiction treatment programs, such as Sierra Tucson in Arizona, have admitted patients into their programs to address addictive Internet use, and many college campuses have begun support groups to help students who feel they are addicted to the Internet (Young 2007).

Anecdotal reports and small-scale open-label studies show benefit from cognitive-behavior approaches similar to the treatment of other behavioral addictions and chemical dependencies. Some strategies suggested by Young (2007) include disrupting entrenched patterns of use by using the Internet at different times from usual; employing external events to force limits on time spent on the Internet, such as appointments or even alarm clocks; setting specific goals for time spent on the Internet, such as 1 hour or less per day, rather than the more general goal of decreasing total time spent; writing cue cards with reminders of both the negative life consequences of addictive Internet use and the benefits of stopping addictive use; writing a list of all the positive life experiences, activities, and social connections that are lost when patients engage in addictive Internet use; and employing support groups and family therapy. An open-label study by Young (2007) of 114 Internet-addicted individuals treated at the Center for Online Addiction showed that at 6 months' follow up, subjects treated with CBT were better able to manage their Internet use; reported improved motivation to stop abusing the Internet; and demonstrated improved ability to control their computer use, function in offline relationships, abstain from online sexual material, engage in offline activities, and maintain abstinence from problematic Internet applications.

Studies examining pharmacological treatments for Internet addiction disorder mainly focus on treating comorbid psychiatric conditions such as major depressive disorder, generalized anxiety disorder, and ADHD. Selective serotonin reuptake inhibitors (SSRIs) have demonstrated some positive effect (Arisoy 2009; Atmaca 2007; Huang et al. 2010; Sattar and Ramaswamy 2004; Wieland 2005). One study by Dell'Osso et al. (2008) treated 14 subjects for a primary diagnosis of impulsive-compulsive Internet usage and found a mean decrease in Internet use from 36.8 hours/week to 16.5 hours/week. A study by Han et al. (2010) found bupropion to be helpful in decreasing craving for Internet video game play, total game play time, and cue-induced brain activity in the dorsolateral prefrontal cortex after 6 weeks of medication treatment. In addition to multiple case reports of successful use of SSRIs, mood stabilizers, and atypical antipsychotics combined with SSRIs (Atmaca 2007; Sattar and Ramaswamy 2004; Shapira et al. 2000), there is a case report of Internet addiction treated successfully with naltrexone (Bostwick and Bucci 2008).

Clinical Issues in This Case

David represents a complicated but common presentation of Internet addiction because his addictive behavior is intertwined with several other psychiatric issues, and it is unclear whether Internet addiction is a primary clinical diagnosis or a secondary manifestation of his depression, anxiety, ADHD, OCD-like syndrome, or attempt to self-medicate intensely negative mood states. However, this conundrum is not so different from diagnosing in the face of other addictions, both behavioral and chemical, that could be manifestations of other psychiatric disorders, and many would argue that self-medication is a part of most addictive behaviors. In this author's opinion, the fact that there are other comorbid clinical conditions does not negate the fact that David meets all of the most basic criteria for all addictions: tolerance, withdrawal, loss of control, and continued and escalating use despite increasingly negative consequences (American Society of Addiction Medicine 2011).

Although the psychotherapeutic approach to addressing David's Internet addiction is similar to therapy for other addictions, including motivational interviewing and individually tailored CBT, David's pharmacological management is quite complicated. Deciding whether to conceptualize Internet addiction as a primary dysfunction of the reward system, a self-medication for anxiety or depression, or an OCD-spectrum illness has important implications for the pharmacological approach to the patient's treatment. In addition, the treatment of ADHD with stimulants has the potential to exacerbate anxiety and obsessional mental processes.

In David's case, the first step was to address the patient's anxiety, which could also have been a symptom of his ADHD as well as a cause of self-medication with the Internet. Treatment with an SSRI had an excellent effect on his anxiety, but it had little effect on his concentration or on the frequency and length of time he spent on the Internet. On the other hand, stimulant medication had an excellent effect on David's ADHD symptoms but increased his anxiety and worsened his work performance. However, stimulants, as well as dopaminergic recreational drugs, tend to worsen obsessive and compulsive behaviors, as was seen in David's case (Han et al. 2009). Thus, treatment with stimulants was important specifically for the treatment of David's ADHD, but it worsened his overall clinical picture because it intensified his compulsive sexual use of the Internet. Changing treatment for ADHD to a nonstimulant medication was the only viable way to address this component of David's overall clinical picture. Use of the SSRI in combination with a low dose of an atypical antipsychotic and a low dose of a slow-release benzodiazepine—a common combination for the treatment of OCD—seemed helpful for many of David's symptoms. Nonetheless, David's compulsive Internet use returned. It is unclear whether this is because the medication treatment was not targeting the primary clinical issues or because Internet use, which may have begun as self-medication for his other conditions, eventually became its own independent condition requiring the classic psychotherapeutic treatment of addictions with motivational interviewing and CBT. In fact, it was the combination of both the pharmacological and the psychological interventions that brought about the most dramatic and longest-lasting improvement. Unfortunately, a necessary change in David's medication due to cost resulted in a loss of his clinical improvement, and he was lost to treatment. David's case illustrates both the complexity of treating Internet addiction and the importance of treating all of the comorbid conditions simultaneously.

Key Points

- Internet addiction is a behavioral syndrome that demonstrates many of the fundamental characteristics of other behavioral addictions such as tolerance, withdrawal, loss of control, and continued use despite negative consequences.
- Internet addiction is a syndrome that is seen with increasing frequency and severity as use of the Internet proliferates and more individuals are regularly exposed to it.
- Internet behavior follows the classic behavior model of variable intermittent positive reinforcement, which can lead to compulsive repetition of a learned behavior, even more than with consistent positive reinforcement, resulting in an even stronger compulsion to repeat the behavior.

References

American Psychiatric Association: Diagnostic and Statistical Manual of Mental Disorders, 5th Edition. Washington, DC, American Psychiatric Association, 2013

American Society of Addiction Medicine: Public Policy Statement: Definition of Addiction. Chevy Chase, MD, American Society of Addiction Medicine, 2011. Available at: http://www.asam.org/for-the-public/definition-of-addiction. Accessed October 20, 2013.

Arisoy O: Internet addiction and its treatment. Psikiyatride Guncel Yaklasimlar 1:55–67, 2009

Atmaca M: A case of problematic Internet use successfully treated with an SSRI-antipsychotic combination (letter). Prog Neuropsychopharmacol Biol Psychiatry 31:961–962, 2007

Bai Y-M, Lin C-C, Chen J-Y: Internet addiction disorder among clients of a virtual clinic (letter). Psychiatr Serv 52:1397, 2001

Bostwick JM, Bucci JA: Internet sex addiction treated with naltrexone. Mayo Clinic Proc 83:226–230, 2008

Caplan SE: Problematic Internet use and psychosocial well-being: development of a theory-based cognitive-behavioral measurement instrument. Comput Human Behav 18:553–575, 2002

Chakraborty K, Basu D, Kumar K: Internet addiction: consensus, controversies, and the way ahead. East Asian Arch Psychiatry 20:123–132, 2010

Cooper A, Putnam DE, Planchon LA, et al: Online sexual compulsivity: getting tangled in the net. Sexual Addiction and Compulsivity 6:79–104, 1999

Davis RA: A cognitive behavioral model of pathological Internet use (PIU). Comput Human Behav 17:187–195, 2001

Dell'Osso B, Hadley S, Allen A, et al: Escitalopram in the treatment of impulsive-compulsive Internet usage disorder: an open-label trial followed by a double-blind discontinuation phase. J Clin Psychiatry 69:452–456, 2008

Demetrovics Z, Szeredi B, Rozsa S: The three-factor model of Internet addiction: the development of the Problematic Internet Use Questionnaire. Behav Res Methods 40:563–574, 2008

Dowling NA, Quirk KL: Screening for Internet dependence: do the proposed diagnostic criteria differentiate normal from dependent Internet use? Cyberpsychol Behav 12:21–27, 2009

Ferraro G, Caci B, D'Amico A, et al: Internet addiction disorder: An Italian study. Cyberpsychol Behav 10:170–175, 2007

Grohol JM: Internet addiction guide. PsychCentral, 2005. Available at: http://psychcentral.com/netaddiction/. Accessed April 20, 2011.

Han DH, Lee YS, Na C, et al: The effect of methylphenidate on Internet video game play in children with attention-deficit/hyperactivity disorder. Compr Psychiatry 50:251–256, 2009

Han DH, Hwang JW, Renshaw PF: Bupropion sustained release treatment decreases craving for video games and cue-induced brain activity in patients with Internet video game addiction. Exp Clin Psychopharmacol 18:297–304, 2010

Huang X-Q, Li M-C, Tao R: Treatment of Internet addiction. Curr Psychiatry Rep 12:462–470, 2010

Jansen J: Use of the internet in higher-income households. Pew Internet and American Life Project, 2010. Available at: http://www.pewinternet.org/Reports/2010/Better-off-households.aspx. Accessed April 14, 2013.

Khazaal Y, Billieux J, Thorens G, et al: French validation of the Internet Addiction Test. Cyberpsychol Behav 11:703–706, 2008

Ko C-H, Liu G-C, Hsiao S, et al. Brain activities associated with gaming urge of online gaming addiction. J Psychiatr Res 43:739–747, 2009

Lee S: Overcoming Crystal Methamphetamine Addiction. New York, Marlowe and Co, 2006

Madden, M: Internet penetration and impact. Washington, DC, Pew Internet and American Life Project, 2006. Available at http://www.pewinternet.org/Reports/2006/Internet-Penetration-and-Impact.aspx. Accessed October 20, 2013.

McIlvaine AR: Internet addiction: the next disability? Human Resources Executive Online, Feb 28, 2007. Available at: http://www.hreonline.com/HRE/view/story.jhtml?id=9942461. Accessed May 5, 2013.

Meerkerk G, Van Den Eijnden R, Vermulst A, et al: The Compulsive Internet Use Scale (CIUS): some psychometric properties. Cyberpsychol Behav 12:1–6, 2009

Pies RP: Should DSM-V designate "Internet addiction" a mental disorder? Psychiatry 6:31–37, 2009

Saisan J, Smith M, Robinson L, et al: Internet and computer addiction: signs, symptoms, and treatment. Helpguide.org, 2013. Available at: http://www.helpguide.org/mental/internet_cybersex_addiction.htm. Accessed April 14, 2013

Sattar P, Ramaswamy S: Internet gaming addiction. Can J Psychiatry 49:871–872, 2004

Shapira NA, Goldsmith TD, Keck PE Jr, et al: Psychiatric features of individuals with problematic Internet use. J Affect Disord 57:267–272, 2000

Stewart CS: Obsessed with the Internet: a tale from China. Wired, Feb 2010. Available at: http://www.wired.com/magazine/2010/01/ff_internetaddiction. Accessed April 13, 2013.

Tanenbaum AS: Computer Networks. Upper Saddle River, NJ, Prentice Hall, 1996
Tao R, Huang X, Wang J, et al: Proposed diagnostic criteria for Internet addiction. Addiction 105:556–564, 2010
Weinstein A, Lejoyeux M: Internet addiction or excessive Internet use. Am J Drug Alcohol Abuse 36:277–283, 2010
Widyanto L, Griffiths MD, Brunsden V: A psychometric comparison of the Internet Addiction Test, the Internet-Related Problem Scale, and self-diagnosis. Cyberpsychol Behav Soc Netw 14:141–149, 2011
Wieland DM: Computer addiction: implications for nursing psychotherapy practice. Perspect Psychiatr Care 41:153–161, 2005
Winkler A, Dörsing B, Rief W, et al: Treatment of Internet addiction disorder: a meta-analysis. Clin Psychol Rev 33(22):317–329, 2011
Young KS: Caught in the Net: How to Recognize the Signs of Internet Addiction and a Winning Strategy for Recovery. New York, Wiley, 1998
Young KS: Internet addiction: symptoms, evaluation, and treatment, in Innovations in Clinical Practice, Vol 17. Edited by VandeCreek L, Jackson TL. Sarasota, FL, Professional Resource Press, 1999. Available at: http://treatmentcenters.com/downloads/internet-addiction.pdf. Accessed June 24, 2013.
Young KS: Internet addiction and wrongful termination. Center for Internet Addiction, December 2006. Available at: http://netaddictionrecovery.blogspot.com/2006_12_01_archive.html. Accessed October 20, 2013.
Young KS: Cognitive behavior therapy with Internet addicts: treatment outcomes and implications. Cyberpsychol Behav 10:671–679, 2007
Young KS: Clinical assessment of Internet-addicted clients, in Internet Addiction: A Handbook and Guide to Evaluation and Treatment. Edited by Young K, Nabuco de Abreu C. Hoboken, NJ, Wiley, 2011, pp 19–34
Young KS, Nabuco de Abreu C: Internet Addiction: A Handbook and Guide to Evaluation and Treatment. Hoboken, NJ, Wiley, 2011

Questions

13.1 Taylor is a 27-year-old single male with Crohn's disease who likes to spend several hours each night collecting pictures of sexy women in swimsuits that he posts in his photo blog, often unintentionally staying awake until 3:00–4:00 A.M. Recently, he was reprimanded by his manager for declining work performance and being found napping at his desk. He was referred to psychiatry by his gastroenterologist for depressed mood, and on initial evaluation, you diagnose him with high-moderate ADHD, predominantly inattentive type. The best medication to treat his ADHD would be

A. Methylphenidate.
B. Methamphetamine.
C. Bupropion.
D. Lisdexamfetamine.
E. Mixed amphetamine salts.

The correct answer is D.

Stimulants can increase libido as well as compulsive behaviors, both sexual and nonsexual. In this patient, increasing both libido and compulsive behaviors will likely worsen his nighttime Internet activity. In addition, a stimulant during the daytime may lessen his tiredness and mask the negative consequences of his compulsive Internet use, allowing the behavior to continue and worsen. However, bupropion is not a safe medication choice because of the patient's Crohn's disease, which may cause significant electrolyte disturbances and lower his seizure threshold. The other options are all stimulants. Methamphetamine, although approved by the U.S. Food and Drug Administration for the treatment of ADHD, is highly addictive, commonly causes hypersexuality, and likely worsens compulsions (Lee 2006). Of all the stimulant options, lisdexamfetamine has the most gradual peak serum level and the longest half-life, decreasing its risk of chemical addiction and worsening of compulsive behaviors.

13.2 Michael, an accountant at a large company, has had increasing difficulty meeting the requirements of his job. His reports are consistently late, and recently, he has been receiving increasing citations by his supervisor for poor job performance. A coworker who saw him twice looking at Internet pornography sites reported him to their manager. An information technology staff member examined Michael's computer and found that Michael spent 3–4 hours of each workday looking at Internet pornography. The best first course of action for the manager is to

A. Immediately terminate Michael's employment.
B. Refer Michael to the Employee Assistance Program for evaluation of possible Internet addiction disorder and sexual compulsion.
C. Allow Michael to continue working but grant him 1 hour of Internet pornography viewing time each day as a reasonable accommodation for Internet addiction disorder, according to the requirements of the Americans with Disabilities Act.
D. Ignore Michael's Internet behavior and focus solely on numerical indicators of Michael's productivity.

The correct answer is B.

Internet addiction is gaining increasing acceptance by mental health providers as a real clinical entity. Kimberly Young, director of the Center for Online Addiction and a professor of management science at St. Bonaventure University, says, "As Internet addiction gains legitimacy as a clinical syndrome or addictive disorder, companies who provide access to the Internet may be at risk for similar wrongful termination claims" (Young 2006). She recommends that instead of immediate termination, employers should first consider alternative actions, such as referrals to employee-assistance programs to help employees manage or overcome their addictions (McIlvaine 2007). Although the Americans with Disabilities Act protects employees with chemical addictions, such as alcohol and cocaine, it does not allow employees to actively use the addictive substances while performing their jobs. Therefore, although Internet addiction is not a chemical addiction, it would be unlikely that Michael's manager would be required to allow him 1 hour of Internet pornography viewing time each workday as a reasonable accommodation.

Index

Page numbers printed in ***boldface*** type refer to tables or figures.